What People Are Sayin

IT'S TWINS!
PARENT-TO-PARENT ADVICE
FROM INFANCY THROUGH ADOLESCENCE

"One of the coolest parts about being a mom of twin boys is that I have an escort for each arm."

WITHDRAWN

—Niki Taylor, supermodel

"It's a privilege to be associated with the NBA's Orlando Magic, but an even greater honor for me is being a father to nineteen children, including a set of twins. There's something special about multiples, and they have really brought a lot of joy to our family. Susan Heim's book, *It's Twins!*, is realistic about the challenges of raising twins, but what I like best is that it helps parents to see how blessed they are to have children, especially when they arrive as a twosome! Whether raising twins, triplets, or more, every parent of multiples will find splendid advice and wonderful encouragement in this book."

—Pat Williams, senior vice president of the NBA's Orlando Magic and author of *How to Be Like Coach Wooden*

"As a medical doctor and father of seven, including twin boys, I see firsthand the challenges faced by parents raising multiples. Susan Heim has written a valuable resource that's full of advice from the real 'experts'—parents of twins and triplets. *It's Twins!* should be prescribed for every family with multiples."

—Andrew Smith, MD

"I am a twin. Growing up as a matched pair in the eyes of others can make it harder to develop as an individual. I still recall the competition between my brother and me throughout our childhood. It wasn't until we went to separate colleges that I felt free to be my own person rather than half of a set. In *It's Twins!*, Susan Heim really captures the issues that families of multiples encounter and provides helpful solutions for parents raising twins like me."

—William Shoemaker, president, Foresight Digital Company

"I wish that *It's Twins!* had been around when I was raising two sets of twins along with our two other children! Susan Heim really understands what it's like to raise multiples, and she offers such useful and entertaining advice for tackling the challenges of raising twins. And the stories and wisdom from other parents of multiples come straight from the 'experts' who really know what it's like to have twins. If you're raising multiples, take it from me: You need this book!"

—Dolores Janer, mother and grandmother

"Even though *It's Twins!* wasn't available when my eight-year-old twin boys were babies, I'm thrilled to find that this book still has lots of great material for my family. With sections on raising twins through the school years and adolescence, I'll be using this book for years to come! And I've even found myself going back to read the parts about raising infant and toddler twins because the stories bring back so many memories of craziness and sleepless nights. My house is still a mess and life is still a whirlwind (I also have a ten-year-old daughter), but raising twins has been one of the greatest experiences of my life!"

—Joan Aresco, mother of twins

susan m. heim

IT'S TWINS!

PARENT-TO-PARENT ADVICE
FROM INFANCY THROUGH ADOLESCENCE

bettie youngs books

Inspiring each other with hope, possibility, and courage.

HAMPTON ROADS
PUBLISHING COMPANY, INC.

Cover design by Frame25 Productions
Cover art by Roman Milert, c/o Shutterstock

Hampton Roads Publishing Company, Inc.
1125 Stoney Ridge Road
Charlottesville, VA 22902

434-296-2772
fax: 434-296-5096
e-mail: hrpc@hrpub.com
www.hrpub.com

If you are unable to order this book from your local
bookseller, you may order directly from the publisher.
Call 1-800-766-8009, toll-free.

Library of Congress Cataloging-in-Publication Data

Heim, Susan M.
    It's twins! : parent-to-parent advice from infancy through adolescence / Susan
M. Heim.
        p. cm.
    Summary: "Written by a mother of twins, this complete guide to raising multi-
ples from infancy through the high-school years offers insight and advice from
moms and dads at various stages of twin-rearing. Offers important information on
breast-feeding, education, dispelling myths about twins, and ensuring equal treatment while fostering individuality and combating competitiveness"--Provided by
publisher.
    Includes index.
    ISBN-13: 978-1-57174-531-6 (6 x 9 tp : alk. paper)
    1. Twins. 2. Child rearing. 3. Parenting. I. Title.
HQ777.35.H45 2007
649'.143--dc22
                                    2006038247

ISBN 978-1-57174-531-6
10 9 8 7 6 5 4 3
Printed on acid-free paper in the United States

This book is dedicated to all
of the parents of multiples who
so generously shared their stories,
advice, and feedback.
Their contributions were invaluable
and critical to this book's success.
May they always know
how blessed they are
to have twins in the family!

Contents

PART 2: TWIN TODDLERS AND PRESCHOOLERS (Ages 2–4) 109

PART 3: TWIN KIDS (Ages 5–11) 185

Foreword

by Vonetta Flowers,
Olympic gold medalist and mother of twins

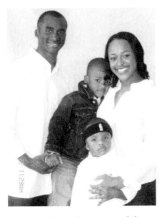

With only four years of experience, I am far from being an expert on how to raise twins. My husband and I have made decisions based on what we thought was best for our family, and we have learned that there are no scientific or canned methods that will prepare you for being a parent . . . especially a parent of twins! In the beginning, I sought the advice of mothers with multiples because I felt that they could speak from experience. Other times, advice was given to me free of charge and without solicitation. Regardless of who was giving the advice, I always seemed to get the typical response, "I promise you, it gets easier!" Fortunately, they were right, but at that point in my life I needed practical advice to help me through the learning process. It's funny how none of the parents were able to slow down long enough to tell me what I needed to do until the "easy" part began. In the end, you'll probably do exactly what I did: You'll make a quality decision based on the information that you have and hope that it was the right one. Having said that, I would like to offer you five pieces of advice that will hopefully better equip you to handle the sometimes chaotic, unpredictable, and wonderful world of living with multiples.

Advice/Tip #1:

Sharing Is Not Just for Kids

Husbands must learn how to take turns. Mothers, let your husband help with the kids. He will truly appreciate you for allowing him to help when you politely nudge him at two, three, and four in the morning to help with the feeding process. He doesn't have to get up every time, but he needs to realize early on that both of you have to work a little overtime for the next few months.

Advice/Tip #2:

Be Honest with People You Trust

Learn how to say yes. If your friends ask you, "Do you need anything?" don't be polite and feed them the typical line, "I'm okay," or "I'll call and let you know if I need anything." Take advantage of the help while it's available. My boys are four now, and at this point there are not many people standing in line to ask if I need anything. Your friends get a warm and fuzzy feeling when they help you out. Early on, they just want to be around the babies, smile, make silly faces, and buy all types of stuff for your children. This type of attention and affection is normal, and you will come to expect this behavior for several months. The good news is that all of this attention may not necessarily come to a sudden end. The bad news is that your list of volunteers may dwindle over time. Therefore, you should spend any free time reconnecting with your spouse while you have people who are more than willing to give up their nights and weekends.

Advice/Tip #3:

Both Children Will Participate in the Baby Olympics at His or Her Own Pace, and Both Will Receive the Highest Reward

My greatest joy as an athlete was when I finally achieved my life-long goal of competing in the Olympics. As a mother, I've seen my children attempt and conquer the greatest challenges in their young lives, and I've been so proud of their accomplishments. There are certain milestones that we as parents celebrate with great enthusiasm. We look forward to the day when our kids grasp their bottles, hold up their heads, roll over, crawl, walk, and—one of my greatest challenges—get potty trained! The "Baby Olympics" will take place for many years, and your young kids will simply amaze you with the speed at which they mature, their strength to continue, and their tenacity to never give up until they've mastered their event. I will admit that it was difficult for me to see one child achieve a goal and not look at the other one and wonder what was taking so long. Even though I knew that both would sit up, crawl, and eventually walk, I wanted them to experience success around the same time. Remember that they are twins and they share a special bond, but they are not clones and will not grow, act, and respond the same way.

Advice/Tip #4:

Use Your Cribs—The Bars Are Meant to Protect Your Children from Falling Out and to Keep Them from Running into Your Bedroom at Night

Allow your kids to sleep in their new cribs. Most parents spend weeks and months preparing the babies' room, and then end up putting the cribs in their rooms or, even worse, allowing their babies to sleep in their beds. This is the first sin. I admit that I was tempted, and I could not resist. After my twins spent nearly two months in the hospital due to their prematurity issues, I felt more comfortable with the boys in my bed. Unfortunately, it took nearly three-and-a-half years to get them out! My advice is to spend the extra money and purchase a baby TV monitor. This will help you in the long run.

Advice/Tip #5:
Remember the Person You Married

It is an absolute must that you spend time with your spouse. If you don't schedule it, then I promise you, it won't happen. And, just in case you're wondering, a family night that includes cartoon characters, singing bears, and pizza typically doesn't qualify as quality time with your spouse. Wives especially need to understand that, for quite a while, your husbands will probably go through withdrawal because your attention will be so focused on the kids. He may never tell you this, but he will have to get used to sharing his wife with—in my case—other men. Spending time with your husband will help your relationship, and he, in turn, will be a better husband and father.

This is my advice to parents of twins, but I want to also encourage you to read *It's Twins!* because it is filled with stories that will inspire, encourage, and strengthen you to get the job done. I spent almost twenty years eating a proper diet, listening to my coaches, and training my body for an event that took less than one minute. I felt that my patience, dedication, and hard work had prepared me for the event, and fortunately, I was right. Now I'll spend the next twenty years training my sons so that they'll be prepared for the game of life. I believe that *It's Twins!* will serve as a wonderful training tool to help you understand the rules of the game, and will also serve as a personal coach that will help you face your toughest and most rewarding challenge . . . raising twins.

Introduction

As any parent of multiples knows, twins are a double blessing— but also a double challenge! What a wonderful gift you've been given to be the parent of multiples! Of course, you know this and treasure your special role, but you've also discovered that life takes on an added dimension of upheaval when your kids arrive as a set. These challenges are unique to those in the "multiples club," and therefore, standard parenting books are often inadequate to address the needs of families with twins (or more). That's why *It's Twins!* is especially tailored for parents, like you, who are navigating the turbulent waters of parenthood with twins. You'll read stories and advice relating to your own unique family situation. You'll be encouraged to really appreciate your very special children. And you'll learn how to handle the extra needs that accompany them.

It's Twins! was written with two important assumptions in mind:

1. Only parents of twins *really* know what you're going through! I've seen parents of multiples literally roll their eyes when other people try to tell them what parenting twins is like. They just don't have a clue! Having closely spaced children is not the same. Parents still have time to get to know the first child as an individual before the second one arrives. And even siblings who are only ten months apart are at vastly different developmental stages when they're

young. The dynamics just aren't the same as they are when you have twins. Therefore, the best advice for raising twins and multiples comes from other parents of twins and multiples. They are the true "experts" in this field, so this book is chock-full of great advice from twins' parents who are walking in your shoes.

2. Parents of twins just don't have time to read long, heavy, and dull advice books! How many times have you bought a parenting book only to let it languish on the shelf? Chances are it just looked too intimidating to forage through when your time was precious. Parents of multiples told me that current parenting books on the market are too dry and "textbooky." Of course, I had to see for myself, so I went to the bookstore and looked at all of the books about raising twins. The parents of multiples were absolutely right! I couldn't imagine having the time or patience to read any of those books, and I resolved right then and there that my book would be different. Parents of multiples let me know that they want quick, to-the-point advice that can be absorbed in a few minutes of reading. They want to be entertained while they are learning. They want tips and suggestions tailored to their own particular situation. And that's what you hold now in your hands—a book that has been organized into lots of bite-sized pieces of wisdom and fun for easy consumption!

How to Use This Book

Not everyone is going through the same phase of life with their twins, so there is no such thing as "one size fits all" advice. Many books on today's market are geared toward new parents and assume that advice is no longer needed for parents of older kids. But that is so wrong! There are new challenges and decisions to be made at every stage of our children's lives, from the first days until they leave the nest. Therefore, this book has been divided into age-appropriate sections so that you know right where to go for the best advice for your family.

Part 1: Twin Babies (Ages 0–1)

Part 2: Twin Toddlers and Preschoolers (Ages 2–4)

Part 3: Twin Kids (Ages 5–11)

Part 4: Twin Tweens and Teens (Ages 12–17)

Just check the table of contents for your twins' age group and jump to the appropriate pages. But, if you do find yourself with a little more reading time, it's also a good idea to read the other sections, too, because they all have information that's relevant to parents raising multiples of any age. Look for these great features:

Twins Tale: These are real-life stories written by parents of multiples about the joys and challenges of raising their kids. Some of them will make you laugh, some will put tears in your eyes, and most will have you nodding your head in agreement. You'll love these stories, whether your kids are one or twenty-one!

Twins Tips: These are quick nuggets of advice for fast and easy reference. They get right to the point in dispensing the best in parenting wisdom.

Intriguing Twins: These fascinating profiles of accomplished twins can be shared with your children, inspiring them to reach for the stars and encouraging them to be proud of their twin status.

Twins Trivia: These informational pieces will dispel some myths about twins and reveal the truths about being a multiple.

Points to Ponder: These guided questions will encourage you to record your own special moments and memories in living life with twins, and they'll help you clarify your thoughts and priorities when challenges come your way.

And, of course, throughout the book you'll find lots of helpful advice from me and other parents of twins. These tricks of the trade will help you get through all the new experiences you'll be having in raising multiples. *It's Twins!* is the ultimate "go-to guide" for all parents of multiples, whether you're a brand-new parent, racing after toddlers, having fun with school-aged kids, or raising adolescent twins. And if you've got triplets, quads, or more, this book has a lot to offer you, too! With lots of common sense, humor, and parental input, *It's Twins!* is sure to put the fun and love back into your ever-challenging role of raising twins. I hope you'll find that it becomes your parenting companion throughout the years of raising your little blessings. And please be sure to send copies to anyone you know who's expecting or raising multiples.

Best wishes,
Susan M. Heim

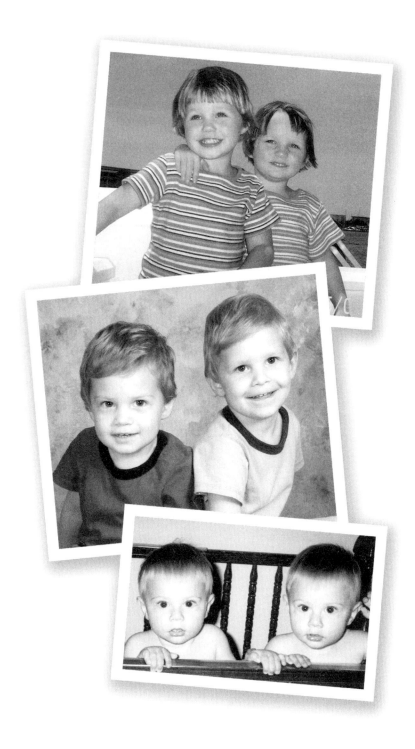

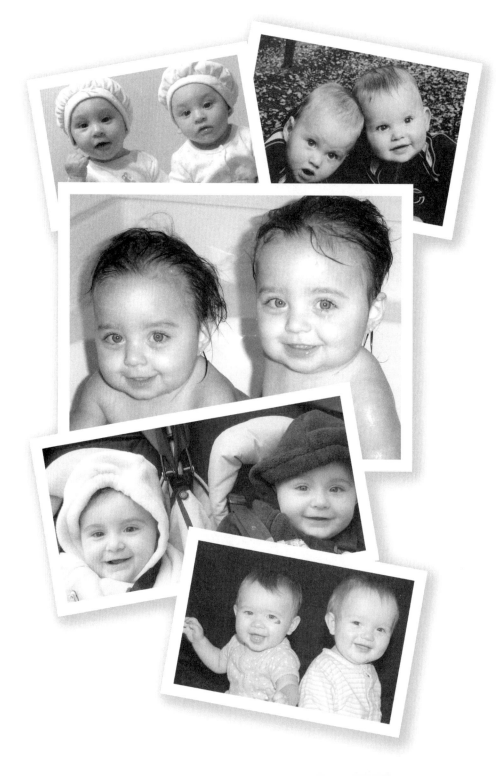

Part 1

Twin Babies
(Ages 0–1)

I just finished co-writing a book called, *Oh, Baby! 7 Ways a Baby Will Change Your Life the First Year.* If I had written that book for the parents of multiples, I would have had to call it, *Oh, Babies! A **Gazillion** Ways Your Multiples Will Change Your Life the First Year!* If you are anything like me, you were totally clueless during pregnancy about what it would *really* be like to have twin babies. And I was already the mother of two singletons. I just didn't get it. My life was totally turned upside down once the twins were born, and I don't think I came up for air for at least six months. It's just too much to comprehend in *theory.* So, if you're expecting twins or multiples now, I'd like to try to prepare you a little better than I was. And, if you're a new parent and currently feel as if you're drowning, help is on the way! Let me assure you that the first year is the toughest, but it will get better. It may seem like three years—or five or ten!—but you will get through it. Every year with your multiples has its challenges, of course, but as time goes on, you'll gain more confidence in your abilities as a parent—and you won't be so affected by sleep deprivation!

Yes, infancy is tough, but it is also precious. Before you know it, you'll be tough pressed to remember the 2 A.M. feedings, the endless diaper changes, and the tandem crying. You'll just remember how adorable your little ones were, and you'll be proud of yourself for successfully navigating the treacherous waters of twin infancy. So, read on for lots of advice from other parents of multiples who have been in your shoes. They have plenty of great tips and stories for getting you through this crucial first year—and even embracing it!

The First Few Weeks

All parents face huge adjustments when they come home from the hospital with new babies, but parents of multiples almost always face more challenges. First, multiples have a nasty habit of arriving a little (or a lot) early, so parents may find that they must leave their tiny babies in the neonatal intensive care unit (NICU) for several days, weeks, or even months before they can bring them home. The constant stress of running back and forth to the hospital several times a day—not knowing if your babies will survive or have complications, worrying about job security and finances, along with extreme fatigue—can make couples wonder if being parents is really the rewarding experience they'd been led to believe it is. Then, when the babies do finally come home, whether together or alone, you're dealing with various monitors, possible medication, worries about Sudden Infant Death Syndrome (SIDS) and your children's health, and round-the-clock feedings with still no sleep. Yes, the first few weeks—and even months—can be an extremely challenging time. All you can do is strive to survive and know that someday your kids will be off to kindergarten and you'll finally have some rest! All kidding aside, it does get better, but having a realistic picture of those first few weeks will help you know what to expect and get through these tough times a little more easily. Twins mom Sage de Beixedon Breslin, PhD, very eloquently explains what her first few weeks home from the hospital were like and how she got through them.

Twins Tale

A REALISTIC LOOK AT THE LIFE OF A NEW MOM
Sage de Beixedon Breslin, PhD

Like lots of Mothers of Multiples (MOMs), my twins came early; maybe not as early as some, but early enough to scare the heck out of me. I've met a lot of MOMs whose babies came at twenty-six and twenty-seven weeks—just at the "age of viability" (which is MOM speak for "a few weeks earlier, and they wouldn't have made it"). Mine came at thirty weeks and four days. When you're a MOM, every day makes a difference when your babies come early. My placenta separated prematurely, and the three of us were nearly lost. Luckily, medical technology scooped us up and dumped us into the NICU. A few days into the process, my husband and I realized how little we knew and how isolated we were. Both of us bemoaned the fact that not a single member of our medical team, friends, or families had prepared us for what *might* (and eventually did) happen with our twin birth.

So, as much as I'd love to just say, "Oh, twins, double the fun!" I can't in good faith do that to even a single expectant MOM who picks up this book. Twins are an incredible gift, and being a good, healthy twin mom requires skills that singleton moms may never have to develop. So, if you're bringing home babies, there are a few things you should consider and digest before the blessed event.

It's time to leave the hospital, but your babies may not come with you. Because twins are often small and underdeveloped when they are born, they may not be able to head home with you when you are discharged. Many times, it only takes a few days for babies to gain their bearings and prepare for life outside the womb. In other cases, it may take significantly longer. For us, we spent a ragged seven weeks in the NICU, and we weren't even sure we were ready for them to come home when they were released.

Many twins who come early aren't able to hold their heart rates steady, so monitors are used for apnea and bradycardiac episodes. The monitors—loud sirens—actually stimulate the babies to breathe and typically correct the problem. As a twin mom, it takes some getting used to—wires and electrodes attached to the babies, monitors to transport everywhere you go, and alarms sounding several times a day. (I figure I got one gray hair for every alarm that sounded.)

Our twins also had to take caffeine (no, it doesn't stunt their growth—that's just a myth) to keep their heart rates high enough. Other babies require additional medications, so we felt lucky that our babies just had caffeine to go home with. I elicited quite a few chuckles from the NICU staff when I asked whether I could have a cup of coffee in the morning. I was told by our neonatologist (who was trying to keep her composure) that I could drink Starbucks all day long and never take in enough caffeine to match the dosage my twins were getting.

Breastfeeding may be delayed. Another issue that may arise for twin moms is that if your babies are born before thirty-five weeks, they may not have the sucking skills to nurse as soon as they are delivered. For some moms, this is not an issue, but for others who seek to bond with their babies through nursing, the delay is heart-wrenching.

I pumped multiple times per day for that month that I waited for my babies to catch up to me. I diligently brought them breast milk, which they received initially through tubes that ran from their noses to their stomachs, and then eventually they were fed by tiny one-ounce bottles. Sometimes I pumped in the NICU next to their crib, just to pretend that I was nursing them. Eventually, nurses taught me how to breastfeed my tiny little guys, one at a time, for nearly forty minutes at a time—to feed just more than one ounce. By the time we left the NICU, the team was proud that I could feed both babies in an hour's time. I didn't realize how problematic that would be until I got home.

Postpartum blues can hit hard. The delays that many MOMS face can also promote the onset of postpartum blues—psychologese for "depression after you've had a baby." While most of us feel a little down as our hormones shift and we acclimate to having a newborn, MOMs face a unique challenge. If babies are not big enough to nurse at the same time, mother may be up all night just trying to get the job done. (You do the math: If it takes forty minutes to nurse one baby, and you've got two, by the time that you've nursed both, it's time to nurse baby #1 again!) Many MOMs end up pumping (which may only take fifteen minutes) and bottling through the night. Others just use formula to make it through the night so they can get a little sleep between feedings.

The first three days after my twins came home, I did not sleep. Between the monitors going off, their crying (the relative silence of their room compared to the noisy NICU apparently irritated the heck out of them), and their non-stop feeding, I couldn't manage more than a few minutes of rest at a time. By day four, I found myself sitting in the shower sobbing hysterically and wondering how I was going to survive. A great friend came to the rescue and told me that she was locking me in my room for eight hours. I could do whatever I wanted, but she wouldn't unlock the door during that time. She slept in the chair in the twins' room most of the night, rising when they needed to be fed or diapered, and was good to her word. After eight hours, I came downstairs feeling like a new person.

My family heard the story and pooled their funds together to hire a night nanny once every two weeks so that I would never again reach that low. She was a lifesaver.

Eventually, my babies, like most others, learned to go longer and longer between feedings, and the nighttime feedings faded away. Soon, your hormones and cortisol levels return to normal, and the depression passes. If it doesn't, seek the assistance of a local psychiatrist and consider evaluation for medication. Your babies need you, so this is no time to try to gut it out if it stops you from being the best MOM you can be.

Long-term sleep deprivation can be dangerous. As I mentioned previously, many MOMs go days without sleep in the beginning as they get used to having twins or more. And, while this is an impressive skill, it's nothing to toy with. The longer you go without sleep or receive insufficient or disturbed sleep, the higher your risk for serious effects on your mind and body. Your family needs you, so when the babies are asleep, *nap!* Even if you only allow yourself to do this a few times per day, it may at least arrest the more serious consequences. The housework can wait, and family members and friends would just love to pitch in with cooking and child care for that first six to eight weeks. Let them! You'll find it to be a lifesaving gift.

Your marriage will be put on hold. In the beginning, it's likely that your partner may feel even more overwhelmed than you do. At a time when you need terrific support just for getting through the day, he may be unable to give you what you need.

Instead of feeling resentful and angry, try making specific requests of your spouse that you think he can handle, even if it's just picking up take-out or buying diapers. If he's not the warm and fuzzy type, ask your mom or girlfriends for emotional support until he's able to pick up the slack in that department. Whether he's low on sleep (if he's helping with night feedings or diapering), overwhelmed by the chaos produced by multiples, or feeling a little underappreciated (husbands can get lost in the transition to parenthood for that first few months!), try not to take it all personally.

After the first few months, when things have settled into place, make sure that you set aside at least one night per week to be *married*! Go on a date, do stuff that couples do, and give yourself a break from the little tyrants. Your babies will love whichever brave soul you leave them with (just make sure they are up to the job!) and will really be just *fine* without you. Remember that partnership is the foundation for family—whether through marriage, extended family, or community. That African proverb could be no truer for families of multiples: "It takes a village to raise a child," much less two or more!

Points to Ponder

If you are expecting multiples, are you surprised to read about how difficult the first few weeks will be? Do you think you are mentally and physically prepared?

If you've already given birth to your multiples, how does your experience compare to the one just described?

What additional advice would you give to new parents of multiples?

At what point did you find it got easier to get through the days and nights with little multiples?

Breastfeeding Twins: Is It for You?

In speaking with many moms of multiples about this book, one of the most requested topics was advice on breastfeeding twins. Surprisingly, many had been discouraged from breastfeeding by the medical community and wanted reassurance that it was indeed possible. I won't lie and say that breastfeeding twins is always easy. It takes a lot of patience, determination, and dedication. But, if you possess all of these qualities (and a sufficient milk supply, of course), I strongly encourage you to go for it! Twins mom Joanne Higgins Ensign wrote the following article about her own experience with breastfeeding, and she offers some great advice if you're considering this option yourself.

Twins Tale
FIVE THINGS I WISH SOMEONE HAD TOLD ME ABOUT BREASTFEEDING TWINS
Joanne Higgins Ensign

I began my quest to breastfeed twins while on bed rest during my pregnancy. Oh, yes, I was going to be prepared! I received a breastfeeding book (*The Complete Book of Breastfeeding* by Marvin S. Eiger, MD, and Sally Wendkos Olds) from a friend and read it cover to cover. Only about four pages were dedicated to nursing twins. The woman in the pictures was smiling; the babies were all smiles, too. I realize now looking back at those pictures that the babies in the pictures were at least six months old and definitely not newborns. When I read the book, breastfeeding seemed so easy, and I assumed this meant that breastfeeding twins would be relatively easy, too. Seriously, I didn't think it would be much harder than nursing a singleton. Oh my, was I wrong! It is joyful, extremely cost-effective, wonderful for your health both in recovery and long term, and has been proven again and again to be beneficial to your twins' health, but for me it did *not* come easily!

Now, I hope I didn't scare you off, because that is certainly not my intention. I loved breastfeeding! I breastfed my twins for eighteen months. Yes, you read that right—eighteen months! Breastfeeding has the most wonderful calming effect that every stressed mother of multiples needs! It helps promote bonding. It was completely worth the effort and the time, but nursing twins requires some serious determination in the beginning. As time goes on, you too will be the happy, smiling mommy with the happy, smiling twins! There were five things I learned along the way that I really wish someone would have told me in the beginning. I had to learn them the hard way, and I hope to save you from the same pain and suffering.

First and foremost, in order to breastfeed twins, you have to make a serious commitment to yourself to try. You *will* want to quit many times! That's perfectly normal. At the start, it is going to take a lot of your time. I had to make a lot of promises to myself to stay motivated: "I will only do this for the most important first week." "I will only do this for the first six weeks." "I will only do this for three months!" At the end of three months, I said, "Okay, I will only do this for six months." After six months (remember that smiling mommy and babies in the picture!), I was willing to do this for as long as my little darlings wanted to. Any amount of breastfeeding you do is a gift to your babies and yourself. It is *not* something to ever lose your mind over or feel guilty about if it is just too much for you to take on. I, for example, never felt super comfortable nursing twins in public, and I chose to use bottles of either pumped milk or formula whenever I was going to be out with my nursing twins. It doesn't have to be a do-or-die situation. You can work with breastfeeding and develop a method that you feel comfortable with. It's okay if it's not the same as other mothers of multiples—and it definitely won't be the same as a mother of a singleton.

Second, you need to be realistically prepared. Don't kid yourself as I did. This is going to be a challenge, but you can do it! Many people, doctors even, will tell you not to even try breastfeeding twins or that it is not possible. Others will tell you that you shouldn't supplement with formula or ever, ever use a bottle. The truth is, you may and probably will need to use bottles and some formula, especially with newborns! Personally, I would have died in the first six weeks without many formula-assisted bottles. And I wasted a lot of time and energy feeling guilty about it. Any newborn is very, very hungry, and newborn twins are just ravenous. I know there are women out there who can make enough milk right away. I read all about a mother of triplets who entirely breastfed for the first five months, but personally, I could not produce enough milk the first few weeks to get my babies nice and full. My babies needed to nurse every ninety minutes to two hours around the clock. I also really wanted to sleep more than ten minutes and have a shower at least once a week. When I came home from the hospital, I tried to completely breastfeed, and while I was making tons of milk for one baby, it took my body a little bit longer to make enough for two. The first compromise I found was to use formula for every other feeding. I breastfed one baby and had someone give a formula bottle to the other one. Then I switched. Those little amounts of formula allowed me to get just a little more much-needed sleep, take a shower, and let my husband and the grandparents help out with some of the many feedings. But, after my husband returned to work and all the grandparents left after just a few short weeks, I was all alone for the first time with my twins, and trying to both breastfeed and bottle feed all by myself was making my life way too complicated. It was just a heck of a lot easier to get both babies nursing at the same time. I wish now I had practiced nursing both babies at the same time while I had so much help around. I still would have needed supplemental formula and bottles so that I could have slept for two straight hours or showered, but I had to learn to tandem nurse all by myself.

That leads me to point number three. Now, please take a *deeeeeep* breath. You are going to have to learn to tandem nurse your twins! That means both babies will be nursing at the same time. If you don't tandem nurse, your other breast is just going to let down milk anyway, and you will end up sopping wet and wasting your precious milk. The alternative, if you are alone, is to nurse one baby while the other baby cries with hunger. If you don't tandem nurse at least some of the time, you will also have to double your time commitment to nursing your hungry babies. That's a lot of time spent nursing, especially if you already have other children. I found it much better to nurse both babies at the same time and have more time to *sleep*! Tandem nursing is tricky in the beginning because both you and your babies are learning how to become a nursing team! In the hospital, it took *two* nurses to make my first tandem nursing session happen. But once mastered, it is well worth the initial effort. You are going to need lots of help the first several times. This can be a really great time for dads to help. Get comfortable and stack up lots of pillows until they're even with your breasts. Your back will kill you if you get into the bad habit of leaning over your babies. Always bring the babies up to you! I suggest you start off with the "football position." This is where the head is forward and the babies' feet point toward your back. Hold one baby very close to your side. Get the baby latched on and ask for help with the second one, doing the exact same thing on the other side. Ask someone to stay close to you in case one baby decides to let go or needs to burp halfway through. I promise you that as the babies grow, this will get much easier. In no time, you will be scooping up babies with one hand and burping while the other one finishes up. It just takes time and practice. Remember to relax and savor the moments. You get to look down at your two beautiful babies. You are blessed. As your babies grow bigger, you can experiment with other positions. My twins loved one in football position and one across. Then they could touch each other while nursing.

I was originally told by the hospital experts to have the babies switch sides halfway through each feeding because sometimes one breast will make a little more milk than the other side and you want to make sure both babies always get plenty to eat. I found this nearly impossible to do. I was just happy to get both babies latched on at the same time! So, I just switched sides after each feeding session. Each baby nurses a little differently and this also helps with the inevitable nipple tenderness, too. I must add that there will be times that you simply cannot tandem nurse. One of your babies may go through a growth spurt before the other one or may be teething or get ill, and you will want to nurse only the baby who has that individual need at that time. I just found tandem nursing to be the most effective use of my breastfeeding time. I also believe my twins really were comforted by all the snuggly time together. They often held hands while nursing. I still cherish that happy picture in my mind today.

Fourth and somewhat controversially, despite what most nursing specialists will tell you these days, a breastfeeding mother of twins will need a basic feeding schedule. I really did try to listen to the "feed on demand" advice at first, and at one point in being a new mommy of twins I did not sleep for twenty-four hours. The schedule I used is what I call "sort of on demand." If one baby gets hungry, at least try to get the other one nursing at the same time, even if it means you may have to wake up a sleeping baby. If you can get them eating together, then they will hopefully also start to fall into a wonderful sleep together. I found that if my babies ate at the same time, they ended up being awake at the same time, and also slept at the same time. It just helped us all start getting into a regular pattern together. The one thing about babies is that their patterns do change quickly. At first it's eat and sleep, and that's about it. Then it becomes play, eat, and sleep, or some combination of the three. The babies are always giving up sleep and adding more time to be awake. The only way to keep them doing all these fantastic things at around the same time throughout the day and night is to feed them at the same time.

Fifth and finally, you must invest in the best darn breast pump that you can afford. It *must* be a double, which is one that can pump both sides at the same time. Once you are a pro at tandem nursing, you will not want to waste any more time only pumping one side at a time. Pumped breast milk means sweet freedom for the mommy! You will need it, and you deserve it! Nothing makes a nursing mommy happier than a freezer full of frozen breast milk. When your freezer is full, you can get your nails done, take a shower, go out for a quick dinner with your mate, return to work, or let the daddy have a chance at trying to figure out how to bottle feed two crying babies at the same time.

Now figuring out *when* to pump can be a little elusive. I asked my doctor in the hospital when I should pump and he said, "Ahhhhhh, after." I said, "Ahhhhhh, after what?" And he said, "After one has nursed, pump the other side," and then he left my room in a hurry. I turned to my mom and said, "But what if the other baby drank all of that side? When exactly am I supposed to pump?" No one would or could answer this question for me. In the beginning, my babies were making sure I was empty all the time. I had no time before or after—or an extra side to pump! I learned that since you are feeding more than one, you will hardly ever have that spare full breast to pump after a nursing session, so you simply will not have as many opportunities to pump. You have to create them if you want spare milk. My first opportunity for really stocking up my freezer came when my babies began sleeping for more than two hours at a time each night. Essentially, they gave up their first late-night feeding, and I then started pumping at night on both sides for about ten minutes before I went to bed. That gave me enough time to make more milk for them at their next feeding. Slowly but surely, my freezer filled up! There are other times you can pump, too. You can always pump right before you need to leave your babies. That also can help prevent any unexpected letdown when someone else's baby decides to cry and your breasts don't realize it's not *your* babies crying. You can pump when you return to your babies, and hopefully someone already gave your darlings some of your defrosted breast milk or formula.

If you have returned to the workplace, pump when you normally would be nursing. I returned to work when my twins were six months old and pumped at work for several months. It's great if your work has a nice, quiet private room, but mine did not. I was still easily able to pump both sides at the same time for ten to fifteen minutes and be finished for several hours. I typically nursed or pumped just before leaving for work. (I liked to leave my house with my breasts empty! As I hinted before, any crying baby caused me a lot of problems!) Then, I pumped around my lunchtime, and I sometimes had to pump again before heading home, depending on my day and schedule. I did try to avoid that so I could nurse again when I got home. I also sometimes got home and my babies hadn't been able to wait for me, and then I needed to pump as soon as I got home. You basically pump anytime you miss a feeding session. Of course, if you have to return to work when your twins are younger, you'll have to pump more often to keep your milk flow strong. Also, know that just because you go back to work doesn't mean you have to completely give up nursing. Your body is amazing and will adjust to your schedule even if you do choose to replace a few feeding sessions with formula because you find it impossible to pump at work. At the end of my breastfeeding experience, I didn't even need to pump at work at all. I nursed in the morning and again at bedtime, and later on, only at bedtime. My body made each small adjustment all on its own.

Before you know it, your multiples will be introduced to all kinds of tasty baby foods, and your time together nursing will eventually end forever. You will find as you look back that the time you spent nursing your twins was precious and that it just flew by. You'll be so glad you gave it a try. I wouldn't have missed it for the world.

Twins Tips
MAXIMIZING THE BREASTFEEDING EXPERIENCE

Get support. Don't hesitate to ask your husband, mother, or friends for help until you feel comfortable doing things on your own. If you have a supportive pediatrician, don't be shy about asking questions. Seek out other mothers who have successfully nursed twins. (You may be able to find them through a local multiples group or an online support group.) Consider contacting the La Leche League or a lactation consultant if you're having problems. Your hospital or doctor can provide you with contact information for these. Make your preferences for breastfeeding versus bottle feeding known to your doctors and the hospital before you give birth so they can support you in your efforts. If they are not supportive, you may want to consider changing doctors or hospitals. (See Christine Scheeler's story for her in-hospital breastfeeding experience.)

Be organized. When you're sleep deprived, it's difficult to remember when you last nursed, which baby nursed on which side, and how long each nursed. Keep a running log with this information, plus a record of wet and soiled diapers. This may be especially important if your twins are premature and your doctor has instructed you to weigh your twins and record bowel movements to make sure they're getting proper nourishment. This information is also helpful if others will be giving the twins a bottle of breast milk or formula.

Take care of yourself. For optimum milk supply, drink lots of fluids (especially water, not soda!), eat healthy foods, and get as much sleep as possible (easier said than done, I know). Don't wear yourself out by trying to keep up with cleaning and cooking. Let others help you out or let it go for a while. You're the only one who can nurse your twins; anyone can do the housework. Make sure you check with your physician before taking any medications or alcohol that might be passed on to your babies.

Be persistent. When you're dealing with the hormonal seesaw of emotions that follow childbirth, it's easy to get frustrated or to break down in tears. It's okay to wallow for a bit, but don't give up! Many mothers report that it takes a while before breastfeeding becomes second nature. Give yourself and your babies an adequate adjustment period.

Change the program for preemies. Premature twins may have difficulty with sucking and swallowing. Don't be distressed if you have to pump your breast milk for a while until your babies are ready to take your breast. Says mother Lorelei Capuzzi, "Born nearly six weeks premature, Rocco and Peter spent two weeks in the NICU where every three hours I attempted to put each one to the breast with no success. So, after each session I returned to my room to pump, and I continued bottle feeding them the expressed breast milk. After nearly four weeks, Rocco eventually mastered breastfeeding, but it took nearly six weeks of diligently continuing this process with Peter before he got the hang of it. Despite these shaky beginnings, I was able to nurse both of my children successfully for thirteen months."

Change the scenery for older babies. Babies more than six months old may begin to get distracted by the sights and sounds of the world around them. You may need to find a quiet place to nurse them, such as a darkened bedroom. Avoid nursing in front of the TV or in a room with lots of activity.

Twins Tale
BREASTFEEDING IN THE HOSPITAL
Christine Scheeler

Prior to delivering my twins, I visited my local La Leche League (LLL). I knew, due to financial reasons, that I really needed to breastfeed my twins exclusively. Upon attending these meetings and seeing many brave women showing their boobs, I gained a true appreciation for the art of breastfeeding. In fact, no longer was breastfeeding something I *needed* to do; it was something I *wanted* to do!

I am the type of person who, when faced with a challenge, reads everything on the subject and thoroughly prepares for that challenge.

Breastfeeding twins was no different. I read breastfeeding book after breastfeeding book. If it was about breastfeeding, I read it.

I also read many books about twins and multiples pregnancies. One of the main facts I noticed in reading these books was that breastfeeding twins was encouraged, but not expected. It seemed that formula would also be a part of our lives. I went to my local LLL meetings each month and continued listening to the stories.

I soon entered the final phase of my pregnancy. The nursery was painted, baby clothes were washed, and the bedding was in place. All was ready for the babies, but I had purchased no bottles. All I had was the one pack of Avent bottles that had been given to us. I kept these as my "emergency, just in case" bottles.

I was placed in the hospital early for bed rest due to swelling. To pass the time, I continued reading more books about breastfeeding. I also attended a breastfeeding class at the hospital where I was to deliver my twins, and I was told to call the lactation department with any questions. That turned out to be a big mistake, as they were very discouraging about nursing newborn twins—especially premature ones.

My sister, Cat, was (and still is) my breastfeeding rock. She, after all, had trudged through the breastfeeding battle before, albeit with a singleton. I knew my sister would help me find the courage to persevere. "Just remember that you want to succeed," she said.

Two days later, my swelling had increased and the protein in my urine was sky-high. There was to be no more waiting. The twins were coming that day.

Since the twins were going to be delivered early, we had many hospital room visits from neonatologists, postpartum nurses, and even my perinatologist. I remember stating very clearly my wish that the babies *not* receive formula if at all possible. I also remember the dejection I felt every time they kind of chuckled and said there are not many moms who can breastfeed twins. If I hadn't already been checked in to deliver my twins, I might have packed my bags and run from the supposedly breastfeeding-friendly hospital!

Since I delivered at thirty-five weeks and five days, both twins were sent to NICU right after delivery. When I returned from the recovery room, I immediately asked for a breast pump and began pumping. I referred to this hospital pump as "The Beast." This thing abused my poor, sensitive boobs and turned my nipples into swollen, cracked, and bleeding blobs. I also developed a very large nipple that I referred to as my "Cyclops Nipple"! I have to admit, it was rather depressing at first that I was only able to get a drop or two of milk. I requested lactation consultation again. I was hoping it wasn't the same lady who had come earlier; thankfully, a few hours later, Juanita showed up. I could tell right away that she was going to be the answer to my prayers.

Juanita believed in me and my goal to breastfeed my twins. So, instead of taunting me and chuckling, she worked with me and taught me how to successfully latch my daughter on as she was now in the regular nursery. She also gave me suggestions and aids to overcome the pain I was beginning to feel as a result of my swollen, cracked Cyclops Nipple.

We were still in a battle with the hospital, though. Every time we went to the NICU to be with our son, we had to send our daughter to the nursery. Every time she was in the nursery, they put thirty milliliters of formula down her throat! Then, every time we would get her back, she'd vomit all over us. At this point, all I wanted to do was take my kids and get out of this unsupportive hospital.

Unfortunately, my son was still in NICU, and his care was being controlled by neonatologists who would not let him out until he ate so much formula per twenty-five minutes. I had so many issues with this. One, I really did not want my son to be bottle fed. It was important to me that he be breastfed. And two, was it really necessary to have him eat so much? My kids were at decent weights when they were born, so it's not like they needed the calories.

Juanita, the excellent lactation consultant, saw my desperation and met us in the NICU on a Friday afternoon. She worked with us for quite a while to get my son to latch on to my breast. We tried several different methods, and the third try was the charm: He actually latched on in NICU and took a full ten milliliters in ten minutes! This was a major triumph for us.

Even though we had been successful breastfeeding in the NICU, our son was still required to take so much formula per feeding. It was a no-win situation for us. We finally just resigned ourselves to doing whatever had to be done just to get our kids out of the hospital!

Finally, the day after my daughter and I were released, my son was released as well. We were free to do whatever we could with them. By this time, I had pretty much given up on the idea of breastfeeding my son. He was already on the bottle, and I was pretty sure he wouldn't latch on. For a full week, I didn't breastfeed him, except maybe one time a day. I was pumping for him with a hospital-grade pump, and this kept up my milk supply in case I was able to successfully breastfeed him later.

We took the twins in for their two-week checkup with the pediatrician. Fortunately, she was very supportive of breastfeeding and really convinced me that I could indeed get my son onto my breast. She suggested that I try to feed him at each feeding time and then weigh him.

Amazingly enough, after each feeding, his intake steadily increased. All it took was one week. By week three, he was 100 percent on the breast.

I am proud of my babies and me for conquering breastfeeding and proving the naysayers wrong. And, I am thankful to the support system I built before I had the babies (my sister, LLL, pediatrician, educating myself, etc.). Had I gone into the hospital not completely ready for the challenges I would face, I am pretty sure that I would be feeding my children formula today.

In the months following the birth of my children, I had the opportunity again to see the people who didn't believe in me: my perinatologist, the NICU doctors, and the lactation consultant who told me I wouldn't be able to feed my twins until their original due date. To say that they were all stunned and disbelieving at my success is an understatement! It was the best reward I could have hoped for, as well as the fact that my twins have been right on track in weight gain since birth.

If you believe in breastfeeding your twins, you will succeed. Believe in yourself before you have your twins. Once your babies are here, you won't have time to read, study, and ask questions. It's easy to be swayed by others' opinions after the birth of your children. Believe in yourself, your babies, and your ability to feed them because I believe in you!

Points to Ponder

If you are expecting twins, do you plan to breastfeed or bottle feed? How did you arrive at this decision? Have you felt pressure from others to pursue one option or another?

If you have new twins, are you breastfeeding? How is it going? What problems are you having?

What have you found really works for you in terms of breastfeeding, such as a desired position for the babies, a particular brand of breast pump, a certain schedule, etc.?

When Bottle Feeding Is the Best Option for You and Your Twins

When I was born in the mid-sixties, my mother never even considered breastfeeding me. It just wasn't really presented as an option by her doctor. Unfortunately, I became a very crabby baby. I would cry and cry after my feedings, and nobody could figure out what was wrong. Years later, doctors determined that I was allergic to cow's milk, and the formula I'd been taking had this ingredient in it. I had a painful tummy ache after every feeding! Fortunately, formulas are much more advanced these days. They're carefully designed to mimic a mother's milk as closely as possible, and there are many different formulations in case a baby can't tolerate certain ones. With my older children, when they weren't breastfeeding, they seemed to tolerate soy formula best. My point is, if you want or need to use formula, you can rest assured that your baby is getting a very nutritional diet. Many mothers use a combination of breast milk (either through nursing or pumped into bottles) and formula. Others, for various reasons, use formula exclusively. Every mother and child is different, so don't let others make you feel poorly about your feeding choices. It's between you, your doctor, and Mother Nature to decide what's best for your twins. Sometimes Mother Nature just doesn't cooperate. I'm a perfect example. Despite having plenty of milk and a wonderful breastfeeding experience with my two older singletons, I was just never able to produce enough milk to satisfy my twins. I used a combination of breastfeeding and bottle feeding for a few months, but finally gave in to bottle feeding exclusively when it became obvious that my well was permanently dry!

Fortunately, I found that bottle feeding has its advantages. For instance, others can more easily help you feed your babies, which is a great timesaver as well as a wonderful bonding experience for your twins' father and grandparents. Bottle feeding also enables you to have more mobility and spares you the problems of sore and engorged breasts, cracked nipples, ugly bras, and embarrassing "letdowns" in public! Twins mom Kim Rich told me, "For medical reasons, I couldn't breastfeed, but this was a plus, frankly. I was able to feed the twins more with formula and they thrived early on, grew well, slept through the night early, and experienced no immune problems thanks to the new formulas that mimic breast milk. Plus, my husband Bill could bond more with the kids. He even did most of the night feedings since I had an older baby to care for. I felt I was a better mom to my girls because I wasn't so exhausted from feeding them."

Twins mother Anne K. Jacobs, PhD, had a very interesting experience in finally arriving at the decision to bottle feed her girls.

Twins Tale

DR. NEW MOM OR HOW I LEARNED TO STOP WORRYING AND LOVE THE BOTTLE
Anne K. Jacobs, PhD

I had very romantic notions of motherhood when I was pregnant with my twin girls. Among these notions was the assumption that I would breastfeed them with ease. As a clinical child psychologist, I read all the research endorsing the many benefits to both child and mother, so naturally I would breastfeed . . . naturally. After confirmation of my pregnancy, I did what I usually do whenever I'm facing a potentially life-changing event: I went shopping. Soon, the nursery was stocked, complete with a nursing pillow specifically designed for breastfeeding twins and a top-of-the-line breast pump. I also had an assortment of sassy nursing tank tops. I walked in the bedroom to find my husband grinning while he snapped and unsnapped the nursing tanks. "Oh, no," I piously scolded. "These are not for your use. They are for the babies." I read all of the books on nursing multiples and prepared my snappy comebacks should some ignorant stranger make a rude comment if I was feeding the girls in public. Yes, I planned to take the show on the road. What could be more natural than a mother nursing her children? I was ready.

Our two little beauties arrived at thirty-two weeks by emergency C-section. Sarah weighed in at 2 pounds, 5 ounces, while Keegan topped the scales at a whopping 3 pounds, 6.8 ounces. While they were in the NICU, I diligently used the pump to ensure that my milk supply would not falter. Sure, the pump did not exactly fit into my romanticized picture of feeding my girls, but I reminded myself that it was temporary. Soon the girls were strong enough to practice latching on. My husband and I were already doing "kangaroo care," where we cuddled the girls, skin to skin. Both Sarah and Keegan had begun to root, so I was eager to begin practice. The NICU staff did their absolute best to create a calm, private environment for this process. Nonetheless, we were still in a room with up to five other families and many beeping monitors. To make matters worse, somehow every priest and chaplain seemed to know when we were practicing breastfeeding and chose that moment to peek around the curtain to offer their blessings. I'm not a shy woman, but the interruptions were distracting. There were a few times when the girls latched on successfully, but it wasn't long enough to offer them any nutrition.

After four weeks, the day arrived when Keegan was ready to go home. The breastfeeding had not gone well, but I had a meeting scheduled with the lactation consultant prior to Keegan's discharge from the hospital. Our hospital has a wonderful rooming-in program where we stayed overnight in a mini-suite with our new baby as a prelude to flying solo. There we were—my excited husband, an unsuspecting Keegan, and me—all eagerly awaiting our first appointment with the lactation consultant whom I will refer to as "Ms. Grabby." Ms. Grabby arrived with her bag full of gear and a cheery smile. I assured her that I had already read all of the breastfeeding books and pamphlets. Her smile in response reflected something akin to weary pity. Despite several attempts, I was unsuccessful in helping Keegan latch on. She cried and vigorously shook her head from side to side. "Don't worry," said Ms. Grabby, "she's just showing a vigorous rooting reflex. This is good." "Really?" I asked. "Because to me, it looks like she is strongly indicating something more along the lines of, 'No, no, *no*, Mommy!'" As if feeling rejected by one's child in front of an audience isn't embarrassing enough, Ms. Grabby then reached out and grabbed my breast. "Here, let me help you get started," she explained. Squeeze! Now I was feeling as though we should at least be on a first-name basis. "So, do you like long walks on the beach, too?" I asked, but she was undeterred in her mission. Ms. Grabby helped position my breast and Keegan's head. Once again, my little one tearfully shook her head no, no, no. She never latched on. For something so natural, this process was proving tricky.

Finally, Ms. Grabby suggested that we use a combination of a nipple shield with a syringe and tube. The idea is that the shield would fit over my nipple, holding a small supply of milk so that Keegan would receive immediate gratification. She explained that we would fill the syringe with breast milk, which would be gently pushed down the tube and into the nipple shield. Keegan was then expected to latch on to the plastic shield and begin to approximate nursing. So, now I was supposed to position my baby's head, secure the shield, hold up the syringe, and distribute the milk (with only two hands, mind you), all the while providing a calm, nurturing experience for Keegan? This was not feeling natural. This was feeling like I was part of the special effects crew on a science fiction movie. I did what every mature, hormonal, postpartum woman would do at this point—I refused further assistance, proclaimed that we would sort this out at home, and tried not to cry all over my strong façade. At least the experience was not a total loss. When concerned others asked how the session went, my husband replied, "Great! I got to see a woman get to second base with my wife, *and* it was covered by insurance!"

Sarah came home two weeks after her younger sister. I had been told that having both girls home would help with the breastfeeding and my milk production. Neither girl could latch on well and both quickly grew frustrated, as did I. I wanted to give the girls breast milk to aid their development, but I did not want feeding times to be stressful for them. The priority, after all, was that they put on weight, so I surrendered to the pump. Pumping was another experience altogether. Nothing illustrates motherhood like sitting at a table alone at 3 A.M., pumping milk while looking at a picture of your babies. The experience wasn't working for me. My milk supply seemed to have reached a plateau, and I felt inefficient. I began propping the collection bottles against the table and reading crime novels or writing thank you notes as I pumped. While the La Leche League does not specifically recommend reading about murders, it did not reduce my milk production. I was stressed out. I was depressed. I was beyond tired. I found myself crying over the pages of the *Diagnostic and Statistical*

Manual of Mental Disorders, 4th Edition. "If I don't meet the criteria for postpartum depression, why do I feel so bad?!" The answer was simple. Being premature, my girls took thirty minutes to finish their meager amounts of milk. They had to then be held upright for another thirty minutes to help counter the reflux problems. Afterward, I would retreat to the kitchen to pump and wash bottles—approximately thirty minutes. If you do the math, that comes out to one-and-a-half hours of feeding-related activities in each three-hour feeding cycle; and that is assuming that nobody throws up and I'm on cleanup duty. This is why I was feeling— excuse the clinical term—crappy.

Now would be a good time for me to talk about my feelings. No, not my emotional feelings, but rather, what it felt like physically to be a human dairy queen. I enjoyed having fuller breasts (any added inches to a lifelong A cup can make one feel like a glamorous porn star), but that was about it. I did not like the physical discomfort that came from being away from my daughters for even a couple of hours. I absolutely despised feeling tethered to the pump. I certainly did not like the leaking. During the pregnancy, I gave up certain illusions of control, but now that the girls were born, I was expecting to be back in control of my own body at least. Not only could I not control when my milk would let down, but I found I couldn't coax my body to produce enough milk for my girls. I could have handled the unpleasant side effects if I had been effective at breastfeeding. I had no excuses. I had a very supportive husband, my parents were nearby to help out in every way possible, and I had wonderful resources through our hospital. Despite dubbing her "Ms. Grabby," I did receive a lot of helpful information from the lactation consultant. The way I saw it, I had no excuse to fail, yet I did.

On a positive note, Sarah and Keegan were growing like weeds. Soon we did not have to roll up the sleeves on their preemie clothes. They were growing, and they were hungry. Unfortunately, my body was not cooperating. I rarely take medication, but out of desperation I asked my obstetrician to prescribe a medication to increase my milk supply. I took it religiously, but there was no change for the better. On top of it all, I was feeling worse emotionally. I checked out the side effects of the pills and found that they may result in feelings of depression and anxiety. The advice I received from doctors and family members was to give what little milk I could produce to Sarah because she was smaller. When looking at my two babies, however, I couldn't bear the idea of choosing one over the other despite the inherent logic in doing so. One afternoon while I was pumping away and listening to my parents take care of my daughters in the next room I had a moment of clarity. I decided then that I would stop putting my time and energy into a task at which I was failing and instead focus my resources on what I did have to offer my girls. My family was supportive, we consulted with our pediatrician, and my husband picked up the formula. I grabbed my first Dr. Pepper in a year and headed into the room to just be present for my girls. I figured that would be a good place to start.

Currently, Sarah and Keegan are healthy, happy nine-month-old girls. They have never had an illness and continue to develop well. Our relationship is more than I thought it would be. We fit together. I don't just love my girls; I thoroughly enjoy being around these two little characters. I did initially feel guilty for not breastfeeding and I continue to admire women who are able to provide for their children in this manner. Over the months, however, I have found that my daughters thrived on what I did have to offer: consistency, patience, and playfulness. In addition to the typical baby-related duties, we spend our days reading, practicing new skills, exploring new things, and setting aside time to be silly. What I have learned in these nine months is that while I walked around with an image of ideal motherhood in my head, life had something completely different and wonderful to offer. My journey to become a mother did not fall into place naturally. After years of trying to conceive naturally, in vitro fertilization provided the answer. After weeks of childbirth classes, an emergency C-section was necessary. And, after almost three months of trying to breastfeed, the bottle was a welcome solution. Despite the invasive medical procedures, all of the technology and contraptions, there was one thing that felt natural. Spending time with Sarah and Keegan and realizing that I do have something valuable to offer them feels like the most natural thing in the world.

Points to Ponder

Were you breastfed or bottle fed as a baby? Why did your mother make this choice? How has this influenced your own choice about feeding your babies?

If you bottle feed your twins, how do you feel about this? Do you feel guilty that you're not giving them breast milk, or do you feel comfortable knowing that your babies are being well fed?

If you bottle feed, what has been the reaction of others to this decision? Have people been mostly supportive or critical?

Twins Trivia

DOES A WOMAN'S DIET AFFECT HER CHANCES OF HAVING TWINS?

According to Gary Steinman, MD, PhD, a specialist in multiple-birth pregnancies, women who consume animal products, especially dairy, are five times more likely to conceive twins. His study was published in the May 2006 issue of *The Journal of Reproductive Medicine.* This may be caused by the presence of insulin-like growth factor (IGF), a protein that's released from human and animal livers in response to growth hormone. It increases the sensitivity of the ovaries to follicle-stimulating hormone, which increases ovulation. IGF may also enable embryos to survive better in the early stages of development. In Dr. Steinman's studies, women who are vegans (consume no animal products) had about 13 percent less IGF in their blood than women who consume dairy products, and they only produced twins at one-fifth the rate of women who eat dairy. Dr. Steinman believes that the introduction of growth hormone treatment to cows to help them increase their milk and beef production may be a factor in the increased rate of twin births in humans.

Twins Tips

CHOOSE YOUR PEDIATRICIAN CAREFULLY
Pam Pace

Take time in choosing your pediatrician. Select one who has lots of multiples in his or her practice. Caring for multiples is so very different from caring for one baby at a time. Many of the rules that apply to a singleton do not apply to two or three (or more!) babies of the same age. If your multiples were premature, find a pediatrician who has plenty of experience in handling preemies. Interview pediatricians carefully and ask them about their parenting philosophies. Make sure you feel comfortable with their advice. And rule out anyone who rushes you out of the office. It takes time to examine more than one baby. You don't want to see a doctor who's in a hurry to get you out of his or her office. Seek recommendations from other parents, especially if you're acquainted with other parents of multiples. Interview as many doctors as necessary until you find one you love! Keep in mind that your pediatrician will be caring for your babies for many years, and you'll want to build a satisfying, long-term relationship with him or her.

Points to Ponder

What qualities do you want your pediatrician to have, especially in light of the fact that you have multiples?

If you've already chosen a pediatrician, what do you like about him or her? Are you displeased about anything? Would you recommend this doctor to someone else?

If you haven't found a pediatrician yet, what is your plan for finding one you're happy with? If you've found one, how did you go about making your choice?

Am I a Bad Parent If I Can't Tell My Twins Apart?

Relax . . . many parents have gotten their twins mixed up! This is especially common when they're newborns and you haven't yet become accustomed to their distinct personalities and mannerisms. (And, they haven't fully developed them yet!) Of course, this problem is most common with identical twins, but even fraternal twins can look alike—especially if you're fumbling to change a diaper at three in the morning! So, don't beat yourself up if you get them confused. You're not going to cause them emotional distress at this age by mixing them up. Of course, if either twin requires medication or some sort of special care, it is important to devise a system for telling them apart until you're certain you know their identities. Some parents leave on their babies' hospital bracelets or anklets for a while. Leslie Kelley-Genson, mom of identical twin boys, suggests painting a toenail. She advises, "This is especially helpful for parents of identical twins because if the babies are naked or just in their diapers, it's impossible to tell them apart. Obviously, this advice only holds until they figure out how to get their toes in their mouths, but by then you should have pretty much figured out who's who anyway." (Don't put polish on their fingernails as they often have their fingers in their mouths from day one!) Leslie continues, "This was also helpful when the babies were left in the care of a third party, so you're not relying on them to remember who is who. We had one episode in which my mom dressed them, socks and all, but mistakenly told us the wrong names. We went on for most of that day thinking Ben was Seth and Seth was Ben, until I was changing who I thought was Ben for bedtime and noticed a birthmark on the back of his leg that I associated with Seth. I took off his socks, saw the painted nail, and realized sure enough it was Seth. The toenail saved us!" Leslie also recommends color coding—dressing each child in his or her "own" color for a while. She told me, "We always dressed Ben in blue, from the little cap at the hospital on up to about age two when he began picking his own outfits. It started as a system to make it easier for strangers (and, yes, us sleep-deprived parents) to tell them apart. But it had a more important, secondary effect that we've since discovered but never would have guessed at the time: Now when I look back at photos of their early years, the only way I can tell them apart is because Ben is in blue and Seth is in whatever color of the rainbow happened to be at hand that day!" Of course, make sure you turn on a dim light if you're dressing your babies in the middle of the night so you put on the correct colors. If all else fails and you still find yourself at a loss to identify them, call your doctor who can match them up with their birth records.

And, just to prove that other parents really have gotten their twins mixed up, read on for Lisa Clifton Philbrook's story of "mistaken identity"!

Twins Tale

THAT'S THE WRONG ONE!!!
Lisa Clifton Philbrook

I am a first-time mother blessed with identical twin girls, Taylor Madison and Haylie Madelyn. Raising them is a lot more difficult than I thought it would be, but I would never trade having twins for the world. When we go out with the girls, my husband and I are often stopped and asked the typical questions: "Are they twins?" "How old are they?" and the infamous, "How do you tell them apart?" Both my husband and I do not think they look *that* identical. I guess it's because we're the parents and we can tell who's who. But that wasn't the case when they were only a few weeks old . . .

When my girls were born on Friday, April 29, 2005, we could not tell them apart just by looking at them. Their only difference was that Taylor had a birthmark on her back. Once we got home from the hospital, the plan was to keep Taylor's hospital bracelet on and take off Haylie's. If all else failed, we would look at their backs for a birthmark.

One week later, we went to their first doctor's appointment. Both girls were doing very well, but Taylor was diagnosed with jaundice, which is caused by high levels of a pigment in the blood called bilirubin and makes the skin look yellow. We were advised to have Taylor sleep with a bili-blanket, which is an ultraviolet-light blanket. The light changes the bilirubin to a form that a baby can more easily dispose of. Four days later, we were to return for a follow-up appointment to check Taylor's bilirubin level through a simple blood test.

Over the next few days, Taylor did very well with the blanket and she began to look less yellow. At the doctor's office, the nurse asked for Taylor. I pulled the baby from her carrier seat and placed her on the table. The nurse pricked her heel, but Taylor didn't cry! This was very odd because my husband and I noticed when they were born that Taylor got very annoyed when the doctors would check her, while Haylie was more laid-back and couldn't care less. I pulled up her sleeve and no bracelet; I pulled on the other sleeve—no bracelet. Oh, no. This couldn't be happening! I looked at my husband as tears filled up my eyes and said, "That's the wrong baby . . . that's Haylie, not Taylor!" I couldn't believe it. I didn't even know my own child. Even though I knew they are identical, I still felt awful.

My husband looked at the nurse and said, "I'm sure this has happened before with twins . . ." Her response was "No!" I felt even worse, and I couldn't stop crying. My husband hugged me. I picked up Haylie and apologized repeatedly for what I had done.

Taylor finally did get her heel pricked, and her blood levels were fine. She no longer had any signs of jaundice. As we left, I contemplated if I should tell anyone about what had just happened. Would someone think of me as a terrible mother for not knowing my own child? On the way home, I called my mother and told her what had happened, and she reassured me that I was not a terrible mother. After all, my daughters are *identical* twins! That day we went home and painted Taylor's big toenail with bright red nail polish.

I've never told anyone else about this incident until now, but I realized that there must be other parents of identical twins who have experienced similar situations, and I wanted to reassure them that they are *not* terrible parents!

Points to Ponder

Have you ever gotten your twins mixed up with each other? If so, what were the circumstances?

How do you feel when you get them confused? Do you feel like a bad parent, or do you take it in stride?

What distinguishing features do your twins have that help you tell them apart?

Twins Trivia
CAN IDENTICAL TWINS BE NOT IDENTICAL?

Even though identical twins share the same genes, they can be very different in many ways. Sometimes they are different sizes, have different likes and dislikes, or exhibit separate personalities. This occurs because human development is not strictly determined by our genes. For instance, if twins share a placenta and one has a "better connection" to the nutrients it provides, this twin may be larger or display other differences. Scientists also speculate that natural chemical changes in our genetic material may affect the way certain genes dominate. This may explain why identical twins tend to show more differences as they get older and don't spend as much time together: Their natural chemical changes affect their development as individuals.

Twins Tips

JOIN A MULTIPLES GROUP
Pam Pace

It's an excellent idea to join a group for parents of multiples. In fact, I recommend that you join every multiples group you can find! During the pregnancy and the babies' first years, you will be hungry for information and support, especially if you're new parents. There is no such thing as having too much support. The second year of your babies' lives, you can narrow it down to the groups you have enjoyed and benefited from the most. Hopefully, you can find some local groups. There are also some international groups, such as NOMOTC, MOST, and Triplet Connection. Check your local phone book or ask your doctor, librarian, maternity hospital, or other parents for referrals.

Points to Ponder

Have you joined a multiples group or attended a meeting? Why or why not?

If you belong to a multiples group, what are the benefits for you as a parent? In what ways could this group be more helpful for you?

Getting Infant Twins onto a Sleeping Schedule

The first six months of my twins' lives is a blur. My husband and I were so sleep deprived that we wore T-shirts labeled "Grump 1" and "Grump 2." Honestly, those first six months felt like six years! It seemed like our babies had a secret pact to make sure that at least one of them was awake around the clock. As soon as one fell asleep, the other woke up. Of course, as soon as one baby awoke, one of us would race to comfort him for fear he would wake up the other twin. Better to have only one awake, we reasoned, so at least one parent could get some shut-eye. In babies' first three months of life, it is essential that they eat every three hours, so this schedule was unavoidable. But by the time they reached six months of age, we knew we had to do something or we would never have tolerable personalities (or a sex life!) again. We finally decided that the only way we could get them on a schedule was for *us* to set the times, *not* the babies. If one of the twins woke up after only a few hours, we decided to let him cry for a while instead of rushing to pick him up. We no longer worried about waking the other twin, and we often found that the dozing twin would sleep right through the crying or else he'd wake up and they'd both lie there "talking" to each other for a bit. Miraculously, it didn't take long before they figured out that we weren't going to come running if it wasn't time to get up and they gave up their cries, either sleeping or playing until they knew we were willing to be available. That six-month mark was a very welcome turning point in our ability to get some rest!

Twins mom Lisa Crystal told me, "Whoever coined the expression 'sleep like a baby' never had babies like mine!" Here's her story.

Twins Tale
ONE MOM'S QUEST FOR REST
Lisa Crystal

When my oldest child—a strapping, full-term singleton—was just one day old, a nurse brought her to me for feeding and then wheeled her back to the hospital nursery so I could rest. But twenty minutes later the nurse reappeared with the bassinet, muttering under her breath in a foreign tongue. She pointed at my caterwauling bundle of joy. "This one you might have trouble with," she said in English. "This one won't sleep."

Truer words were never spoken. Several months later, "this one" still seemed to log no more than eight hours of shut-eye out of twenty-four—and always in dribs and drabs. I tested various sleep-promoting methods advocated by baby experts. The most promising among them: Place the bassinet next to my bed so I could nurse on demand and drift right back to sleep alongside my sated baby. I really wanted this cozy-sounding strategy to work. But was I the only breastfeeding mom who, when roused at night, made a beeline for the bathroom after guzzling fluids all day? Was mine the only baby who—despite valiantly rooting around for my nipple in the gully carved out in our deluxe pillow-top mattress—was unable to latch on to the breast when I was lying down? And, I wondered, didn't anyone else's baby jealously guard her intestinal contents all day so as to violently expel them at night, often prompting a 3 A.M. change of nightclothes, if not a sponge bath?

After several more failed experiments, I found salvation in a battery-powered swing. At first I used it sparingly; after all, I didn't need experts to tell me that babies require human rather than mechanical cuddling, plenty of "floor time" to strengthen their neck muscles, and so on. But rationalizing that I could always pay for therapy later—either physical for my daughter's atrophied muscles, or psychological for her attachment disorder—I willfully became a swing abuser. My daughter spent daytime naps and much of each night indulging her obsession. I'm not sure how much of that time she actually slept, but I do know that my husband and I enjoyed a lot more shut-eye, especially with a white-noise machine humming away next to our bed to drown out the swing's rhythmic clicking. Day after day, night after night, our little swingaholic rested comfortably in that contraption—until she got so heavy that it wouldn't budge when switched on, even with a fresh set of batteries.

Six years later, I came to realize that my daughter's first year had merely set the stage for the ultimate sleep challenge: twin babies. Naturally, before my sons' births my first purchases were two top-of-the-line baby swings—the kind with a cradle attachment as well as a regular upright seat. The cradles turned out to be a waste of money, as my twins had reflux and could seldom lie prone without losing their latest lunch; besides, they rolled around like a couple of sausages no matter how tightly I wedged rolled-up blankets around them. But the swings were fine, and I began propping the babies in them when they were just a few weeks old. The rocking motion did the job—though since they seemed to prefer stillness after a half hour, someone had to remember to flip off the switch.

Overall, my twins were actually more reliable snoozers than my daughter; given the right conditions, they slept longer, more deeply, and more often. The trouble was they didn't sleep at the same time. All night they'd tag team: One would awaken, eat, fill his diaper (a family trait, apparently), protest the clean up, and rock in his swing until he drifted off—signaling the other to awaken and start the cycle anew.

Whenever I could sufficiently focus my bleary eyes, I consulted the twin-care treatises piled next to my underutilized bed. When one awakens, rouse the other, my sources instructed. So at 3 A.M., while the "awake" one howled, I'd slam the closet door, poke the sleeping baby, and even strip off his nightclothes. He'd just furrow his brow and scrunch down in his swing seat in a state of studied unconsciousness. Removing him from the seat and placing him on the floor was futile. Alas, nothing could rouse my sleeping baby in the middle of the night—except, of course, the rhythmic breathing of his twin brother, once said brother had drifted off again after feeding and defecating. At this point

I'd awaken my husband, who would field the next round with a bottle of formula while I lay fitfully in our bed, exhausted but buzzing with a nocturnal manic energy I hadn't known since college.

I moved on to plan B, also recommended by the experts: Sleep when the babies sleep, day or night. Since I had quit my job, this approach seemed feasible, if somewhat complicated by my need to pick up my daughter from school each day. Still, one early afternoon, with both babies snoozing in the double stroller I'd parked in the front hallway, I ignored the sink full of dirty bottles and lay down on my bed. This was delightfully relaxing for about ten minutes, until the postal worker pretended not to see the "Baby Sleeping" sign hanging on my front door and rang the bell. I got up, signed for the package, and opened the box, which contained yet another baby gift from a well-meaning relative.

Not one to give up, the next day, when the boys were tucked peacefully in their swings, I went horizontal again, this time on the living room couch. That was the cue for the rear neighbor's preschooler to rev up her motorized, ride-on jeep. After ten minutes of the vehicle whining its way across their grassy terrain, I bolted up and brewed tea to soothe my jangling nerves.

And so it went. Each day when I laid down my weary, unwashed head, my "quiet" suburban neighborhood came to life. The recycling truck would drop off an oversized bin right outside the babies' bedroom window. A neighbor would feel a sudden urge to crank his motorized hedge trimmer or jackhammer up the old patio he'd been meaning to get to since last spring. Sometimes even the swings' mechanical drone was no match for these auditory insults. And, even when the babies slept through the din, I could not. The disturbances were so frequent, yet so maddeningly unpredictable, that I spent my "rest" time tensely anticipating the inevitable.

Finally, with me weepy and dangerously exhausted, my husband and I defied the experts and devised a plan of last resort. I gave up nursing at night, and we wedged a mattress in the corner of the living room, where he and I slept on alternate nights. The living room sentry had baby duty from 10 P.M. until 6 A.M., while the lucky off-duty parent got to sleep in our upstairs bedroom all night, door firmly shut, earplugs in, white-noise machine humming. Refreshed and recharged, the rested parent would then take over baby duties the following night.

This arrangement worked surprisingly well. No matter how bad a night I endured with the babies, I could get through it—and the following day—knowing that eight hours of blissful, uninterrupted sleep awaited me the next night. I actually felt rejuvenated within a couple of days and we happily followed this regimen for one year, until the babies slept through the night fairly reliably.

The obvious downside—and always the first thing new moms ask about when I share this particular survival tip—was that my husband and I didn't sleep in the same bed for a year. The advantages of this system were difficult to explain to visitors who spied the rumpled mattress in the living room, especially if they had never had one baby, let alone two. But in truth, that bed in the corner may have saved both my sanity and my marriage. Though my husband and I missed the cuddling and companionship of shared sleeping quarters, we agreed that the ability to actually sleep trumped all else. And, as for action beyond cuddling, our arrangement yielded a surprising benefit: There was something deliciously taboo about sneaking into each other's beds for a quickie before the first night feeding.

Now that my twins are seven and my daughter is a teen, it's safe to say that our unconventional sleep aids had no lasting deleterious effects on any of them—all three even still ride our backyard swings. And my husband and I, though we enjoyed unexpected intimacy during our nocturnal isolation, are grateful to again share a bed every night, where we (usually) partake of uninterrupted sex and slumber whenever we want it.

Now if only I could fall asleep without a white-noise machine.

Points to Ponder

Did you ever imagine you would feel so sleep deprived before you had kids? How has this affected your relationship with your partner?

Have you tried to get your twins onto a sleeping schedule? What methods have you tried? What worked and what didn't?

Do you believe in letting babies "cry it out," going to them as soon as they cry, or something in between? What are the benefits and drawbacks of both options for you and your babies?

Be Prepared for Lots of Attention!

If you don't like to draw attention to yourself, don't head out into public with your twins! They are a sure attention getter. And you'll hear the same questions and comments over and over again. Here's how twins mom Rebecca Adamitis describes it:

Now that Owen and Olivia are eighteen months old, we've heard all of the typical reactions to our "ROO Crew" (the R being for older brother and resident clown/rock star Ryan). I've actually gone from being annoyed with the same questions over and over again to having a little fun with them. For instance, the age-old conversation that every parent of multiples will have regarding their accomplishment goes a little something like the following:

"Oh, my gosh. They are sooooooo adorable. Are they twins?"

"Yes, thank you."

"A girl and a boy. Oh, you are so lucky; you got the best of both worlds. Are they identical?"

"Uh, no, actually, they're fraternal." Duh.

"Oh, you know my neighbor's daughter's best friend's sister is pregnant with twins. Was your pregnancy hard?"

"Oh, you know, it was worth it. Well, I see them starting to fuss. I'd better find a place to change some diapers. It was nice talking with you."

Here's how my conversations go now that Owen and Olivia are eighteen months old.

"Oh, my gosh. They are sooooooo adorable. Are they twins?"

"Mmmm. Ryan, just a sec, Mommy's having a conversation, honey. Could you please stop pulling on my pants, showing everyone my ratty old underwear?"

"A girl and a boy. Oh, you are so lucky; you got the best of both worlds. Are they identical?"

"No, actually, my son was born with a penis and my daughter, thank the Lord, was not."

"Oh, yes. Well, you know my neighbor's daughter's best friend's sister is pregnant with twins. Was your pregnancy hard?"

"Oh, you know, bed rest, I had to give myself various shots throughout the whole thing, hospitalizations, infections, preterm labor, C-section. Essentially, it was a walk in the park."

"Okay, well, you enjoy those children. They're beautiful. Bye-bye now. Have a nice day."

Mission accomplished. But wait. There's more. How about this one:

"Wow. Twins. A boy and a girl. And an older brother, about three-ish. Boy, you must have your hands full."

"Uh . . . uh huh," followed by that little nervous laugh we all do when we're trying to be polite and all we really want to do is scream, "Well, *duh*! Get out of my way, lady, so I can get my gallon of milk before the darling handfuls start having a meltdown!"

I haven't quite had the nerve to say, "Yeah, tell me about it. Hey, you wouldn't want to come home and help me scrub poop out of their pajamas, would you? I could really use the help." Or, "You know, a lot of people have said that. Do you have anything more original? To be honest, that cliché is starting to bore me a bit! How about you share with me the secret of how to make everyone happy and get Mt. Laundry done in one stinkin' day?"

Well, as you can see, at times it's difficult not to get impatient! But it helps to have a sense of humor. It's natural for people to be curious about your children. As twins mom Cheryl Maguire found out, they're celebrities! So, public attention is just part of the territory.

Twins Tale

MY LIFE AS A CELEBRITY ASSISTANT
Cheryl Maguire

I always wondered what it would be like to be a celebrity. I imagined it would be wonderful and glamorous. I never really thought about the downside. Now that I reside with two real-life celebrities, I've found that even going to a restaurant can be a major undertaking!

On our most recent trip to a restaurant, a large crowd was gathered outside. The best route into the place was discussed. We opted for the side door since there seemed to be fewer people near that entrance. Quickly, we made our way to the hostess, trying to protect our celebrities. All of a sudden, the hostess noticed them, and the questions began. "Oh, are they twins? Are they identical? How old are they?"

Amazing! I thought to myself. *She managed to hit the trifecta of questions all in one breath!* I quickly answered all of her questions, only to have her respond with the most popular comment, "Oh, a boy and girl. Now you don't need to have any more babies!" I never realized how many people feel that a boy and a girl constitute the "perfect" American family.

I looked at my watch as the hostess babbled on to the other assistant. Celebrities can be very demanding. If they don't get their way, the whole world is going to hear about it pretty quickly, so I tried to move things along. We were finally seated at our table.

I began to feel the stares all around me. I tried to avoid making eye contact. The little boy at the next table was not going to be avoided. Suddenly, he was at our table trying to touch the celebrities. His parents didn't even try to stop him. In fact, they saw it as an invitation to ask questions and make comments. I quickly answered them, "Yes, they are twins. They are six months old. They are a boy and a girl. No, they are not identical." That last question always boggles my mind. Even though I just told the person that they are boy/girl twins, they still ask if they are identical. After explaining some basic biology facts to them, I usually get one of two reactions. Some people realize their question might have been a little silly, and others just look confused. For the confused ones, I just try to smile politely and move along.

After answering the questions, I turned my attention to my celebrities, and the other celebrity assistant and I tried to enjoy a peaceful meal. I noticed that the couple next to us was talking about us as if we couldn't hear them. Soon, their little boy had found his way back to our table.

A waitress arrived at our table, but I soon realized that she was not our waitress. She stated, "I heard about the twins in the kitchen, and I just had to see them for myself." The questions began, followed by the standard comments.

I turned to the other assistant, who nodded at me. We realized that this situation was just not working out. We got the meal to go and quickly made our exit.

Even though it can be challenging at times to be a celebrity assistant, I will admit it can be lots of fun as well. Celebrities can be quite entertaining. In fact, there isn't a day that goes by when they don't make me laugh about something. They are always testing out their vocal cords and trying out all kinds of crazy moves.

Oh, who am I kidding . . . I love every minute of it!

Points to Ponder

What are the silliest or strangest things that people have said to you about your twins?

How do you feel about the attention your twins receive? Is it annoying, amusing, or a little of both?

In what ways are outings more complicated now that you have twins?

Intriguing Twins
MOSES AND AARON WILCOX

Born on May 18, 1772, twins Moses and Aaron were born to Abel and Mary Wilcox in Killingworth, Connecticut. The twins were so identical that even their closest friends and family members had trouble separating them. They were also alike in temperament. If one was sad or ill, the other one became so, too, even if they were apart! As adults, they both served as officers in the War of 1812 and then later became prosperous merchants and manufacturers.

Their personal lives also ran parallel. They married sisters, Huldah and Mabel Lord, and both had nine children. With their families, they moved to Millsville, Ohio, and farmed together on jointly held land. They also sold small parcels of land for the Connecticut Land Company. Then the Wilcox twins made an odd request: They would give six acres of land to the town for a public square along with twenty dollars to be put toward building the first school if the town's name were changed to Twinsburg. Their unusual request was granted!

The twins who did everything together nearly died together, too, only four years after arriving in Twinsburg. A few minutes after Aaron died in his home, Moses, who lived a half-mile away, is reported to have risen up in his bed and exclaimed, "My brother Aaron is dead, and I shall die, too," which he did a little later in the day. The twins were buried together in the same grave, one above the other, in Twinsburg's Locust Grove Cemetery.

A plaque in the town square reads: "In memory of Moses and Aaron Wilcox, the twin founders who gave Twinsburg its name, and this public park. They were unique in that they married sisters, had an equal number of children, held their property in common, were identical in appearance, were taken ill of the same disease, died on the same day, and are buried in the same grave." It also states: "This monument erected as a permanent tribute to the foresight and integrity of the Wilcox twins who dedicated the land for this park and were instrumental in Twinsburg's cultural, religious, and educational growth."

Twinsburg is now the site of the world's largest annual gathering of twins—more than three thousand sets from around the world. Held the first weekend in August, the Twins Days Festival is an occasion for fun, as well as scientific exploration. Each year, researchers and scientists show up to conduct various surveys and experiments with twin participants. Other events include a "Double Take" parade, a twins' talent show, fireworks, a golf outing, and other contests. There has even been a double wedding: twins marrying twins, of course!

Twins Trivia

WHICH WOMEN ARE MOST LIKELY TO CONCEIVE TWINS?

First, women of "advanced maternal age" (as my doctor labeled me unflatteringly) are more likely than younger women to conceive twins. As they get closer to menopause (after age thirty-five), women begin to ovulate more irregularly. Therefore, the chances of releasing more than one egg in a given menstrual cycle are higher. For some reason as well, if women already have children, they're more likely to have twins. In fact, the probability of having twins is three times higher in women over the age of thirty-five with at least four other children than for women under twenty who are pregnant for the first time. In addition, African-American women have a 1 in 79 chance of conceiving twins; Caucasian women have 1 chance out of 100; and Asian women conceive twins more rarely—1 in 155 pregnancies. Finally, when women first stop taking the birth control pill, their pituitary glands kick in with higher amounts of stimulation than usual, so the chance of conceiving twins is greater in the first month off the pill.

Getting Help!

We'd like to think we can handle everything on our own, but it's certainly no sign of weakness to ask for and accept help. In fact, it will make you a better parent by lowering your stress level and allowing you to get some rest. So the next time someone says, "Let me know if I can help in any way," don't give your standard "Sure, I will" response. Let them know what they can do! Does your friend make great lasagna? Ask her to drop some off to save you from having to cook one night. Do you and your spouse need some together time? Don't be bashful about calling potential sitters. Most people are flattered that you want them to watch your adorable twins. Trust me, if they really don't want to, they won't hesitate to turn you down! But I'm willing to bet they'll be thrilled. The following mom of twins has some great tips for getting the help you need as well as cutting down on the expenses of raising twins.

Twins Tips
HELP IS ON THE WAY!
Marla Feldman

- If someone says she would *love* to come and help you out, don't just say, "Thank you." Grab the calendar and ask what day of the week works best and what time. People love to say things; it is another to follow through!

- Do not be afraid to ask for help. Infant twins are overwhelming!

- Pay for any help you can get if it is economically possible.

- Lower your cleaning and neatness standards and invest in Lysol wipes.

- Simple Green gets everything out.

- Bring a shopping bag to the doctor's office and ask for formula samples. Book your appointments for the same day and time. The nurses will get to know you and your babies. I used to leave with cases of formula!

- Google search baby freebies and twin freebies. Sign up for online offers.

- Call the 800 numbers for offers, too. Grandparents can also get offers. I used to call Beechnut and Gerber every week for coupons. As soon as a packet would arrive, I would call again. They want you to buy their products!

- Do not be squeamish about getting things secondhand. After all, we eat out at restaurants and sleep at hotels, and how many other people have used the forks, spoons, and bedding?

- Ask for everything you need. There are many people out there—more than you realize—who are hanging on to baby items that they no longer need. Put out the word to friends and family, and ask them to ask people. This is especially true if you already have a child and now need a second of every-thing. Just make sure that nothing has been recalled and it meets today's safety standards. (Note from Susan: This is a great tip! My husband and I spread the word that we were looking for a double stroller. A friend of a friend sold us a $300-plus stroller for $40, and she had barely used it because her older child decided he didn't like to ride. Two-and-a-half years later, we're still using that great stroller!)

Points to Ponder

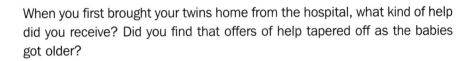

When you first brought your twins home from the hospital, what kind of help did you receive? Did you find that offers of help tapered off as the babies got older?

Have you had to loosen some standards now that you have twins, such as your determination to clean the bathroom every day?

Why are we often hesitant to accept help when we could use it? Have you worried that others won't take care of your children as well as you can?

What kind of money-saving tips have you discovered for your family?

From the Career Track
to the Mommy (or Daddy) Track

Many parents of multiples find that it's more economical to have one parent stay at home with their children than to pay for day care for two or more. At first thought, despite the diminished income, this sounds great. For the parent staying home with the children, there is no more of the 9-to-5 stressors. No more expensive work clothes. No more long commutes. No more unreasonable bosses. Sounds like heaven, right? But the reality is that it's often a greater transition than expected. Now that you're spending your days (and nights) solely caring for twin babies, you have 24/7 stressors! Your clothes are getting ruined from formula stains, and you can't keep your growing kids in clothes long enough to wear them out. Sure, there's no commute, but now you're imprisoned in the house all day. And, instead of one grumpy boss, you've got two babies making constant demands on your time. Add to that, you're not getting financial compensation or words of appreciation for figuring out how to get the twins to sleep at the same time or to surrender their pacifiers. Sure, there are pleasures, but they're sometimes difficult to appreciate when you've had two hours of sleep in the past twenty-four hours.

The transition from the working world to the home front can be particularly painful if you really liked your former job and the career path you were on. It may be a disappointment to know that you'll lose your seniority or won't benefit from all your hard work. Of course, if you were dissatisfied with your job, you may be delighted to finally have an excuse to leave. But whatever situation you're in, think of this stage in your life as a time of new beginnings. It's scary to leave something that's comfortable, but quite often we find that a change is really for the best in the long run.

You may find that, with time, you can have the best of both worlds if you desire. For the first six months of my twins' lives, the only job I was capable of accomplishing was that of nursemaid. Every moment of my life was consumed with caring for my babies and trying to sleep when I wasn't occupied with them. But, once they got onto a more predictable schedule, slowly I began to squeeze back into the working world from home. I contacted a former business colleague who was willing to send me writing and editing assignments on a freelance basis, and my home business was launched. Of course, it took time to build a career at home. I only had nap times and bedtimes to work—and still do! So, naturally, my income dropped drastically. But I was thrilled to be back in the business I loved, and I found that I was actually more productive without the constant meetings and telephone calls that distracted me at the office. Within two years, I had more work than I could handle and contracts for several books—something I doubt I would have accomplished working a forty-hour week at the office. I have the best of both worlds: a career that I love and lots of time with my twins. As my business has grown along with my kids, who are starting to give up naps, I've been able to afford part-time preschool, which gives me more time to write.

Of course, you may be perfectly happy being a full-time parent and not pursuing a career, and that's wonderful, too. You have the most important job in the world—raising a new generation. And that's the best way to make the transition from the workplace to the home place—know that you are important. What you do has huge value, more than being the CEO of a Fortune 500 company or the writer of the next bestselling book. Roxy Ranelli, once an up-and-coming executive before conceiving triplets, finally figured this out, too.

Twins Tale
CLIMBING THE LADDER TO SUCCESS
Roxanne Ranelli

At twenty-eight years of age, I was *finally* living comfortably and quickly climbing the corporate ladder. My main focus in life was to be successful in the workplace. I knew that one day I would have children, but I was not prepared to give up my career and dreams to raise a family. Then I received the news that I was pregnant. At first, I was shocked, confused, and awed that I had to take on this responsibility. I didn't want to believe that I was pregnant, but five home pregnancy tests begged to differ. One of my first thoughts was, "How am I going to work and take care of a baby?"

Once confirmed by the doctor that I was eight weeks pregnant, I made arrangements with local day-care centers to go over the costs and times involved in taking care of my newborn during work hours. Sure, I could stay at home, but I did not want to lose my "place" on the corporate ladder. I was still going to be a career-driven individual, no matter what hand was dealt to me! I enjoyed being the boss and having people look to me for answers. I enjoyed the income that continued to increase over time. I enjoyed having the finer things in life.

Then I was hit with the amazing news that I was having not one baby . . . but three! At that point I had to accept that working outside of the home was not an option anymore. It seemed that everything my world revolved around was going to disappear.

One year later . . .

My children are now six months old and, thankfully, very healthy. A year ago, I felt saddened by the news that my life would change and my career would be put on hold. I now realize that being a mother is one of the greatest and most rewarding challenges in life. I may not have twenty employees looking up to me as their leader, but I have something much more satisfying—three beautiful babies looking to me to teach them about life. I may not have the income that I once desired, but I can say now I am the richest person in the world. Money certainly can't buy love! I may not have the BMW I dreamed of or the house on the lake, but these "finer things in life" don't even compare to the birth of a child. Now when I look back on my desire and drive to work and be successful, I laugh uncontrollably. You see, being a mom is "work." It is more challenging, more rewarding, and more appreciated than any other job you will ever have. And I know that one day I will climb that ladder again. But for now, I have the greatest job in the world and would not trade it for anything.

Points to Ponder

Do you work outside the home or are you a stay-at-home parent? Are you happy with your decision? Why or why not?

If you formerly had a career and now stay home with your children, how have you adjusted? Do you miss anything about going to an office or pursuing a career, or were you thrilled to leave?

Do you think that society values the work of a stay-at-home parent as much as other occupations? Why or why not?

What sacrifices have you had to make now that you're a parent, such as giving up your sports car or postponing vacations? How do you feel about this?

For you personally, is there a way to have a career and parenthood, too? If this is your choice, how do you plan to accomplish this?

Twins Tips
PRODUCTS THAT PARENTS OF MULTIPLES CAN'T LIVE WITHOUT

Lainie Ceasar: The Podee Baby Feeding System saved my life the first year after my twins were born. This self-feeding bottle system allowed me to feed both babies while holding only one. Sometimes I'd put the bouncy chairs on the floor of the kitchen and give both Max and Zack their Podees while I prepared dinner for my husband and me. It was also wonderful when we were on the go. If they needed a bottle while we were taking a walk with the stroller, there was no need to stop. I'd just give them their Podees and we'd continue our shopping or sightseeing excursion.

Lainie Ceasar: The SwaddleMe Adjustable Infant Wrap is a must have for parents of multiples. It was great for the middle of the night when you're trying to swaddle two babies and can barely keep your eyes open!

Kim Rich: Baby Einstein DVDs and videos always calmed our babies down, especially *Baby Mozart*. The classical music and colorful images honestly could stop all crying. (Susan's note: Many parents recommended these videos. My sons' favorites were those with lots of animals, such as *Baby Noah* and *Baby MacDonald*.)

Adarezza Ferrer: The best thing I ever did was to read a book called *The Happiest Baby on the Block* by Dr. Harvey Karp. His five-step approach simulates the womb environment, which helps babies feel better and cry less.

Susan Heim: I love my Graco DuoGlider Double Stroller! When my sons were small, their SnugRide car seats attached right to the stroller, so I could easily transfer them right from the car to the stroller without having to unbuckle them. When they got older, the front and rear seat design made it easier to navigate narrow store aisles, preventing my toddlers from grabbing things from shelves. The large bin in the back carries lots of baby necessities, and it folds up easily to fit in the trunk of my car.

Pam Pace: I found Dreft to be the best detergent for babies' clothing. Also, have a stick of stain remover around as babies' iron supplements and formula can stain clothing. I kept a laundry basket next to the changing table. I also bought a mesh laundry bag with a drawstring for those tiny little socks that our washing machine liked to eat!

Pam Pace: It is very important to love your breast pump! I tried several before I settled in with the Medela Lactino Plus Dual Pump. Go for the best hospital-grade pump available. It will save you time. I was able to pump about seven ounces in about ten minutes.

Potty Training Infant Twins: Is It Possible?

Perhaps you've heard of the potty training method called "elimination communication" or infant potty training. This technique has been used in parts of Asia and rural Sub-Saharan Africa for a long time. The premise is that infants as young as six months old can be trained to use the toilet (or sink or other container), rather than the diaper. (Some experts recommend beginning training even younger, right after babies are born, so they don't get accustomed to using a diaper.) Proponents claim that parents can learn when a baby's ready to "go," through signs such as straining or grunting, and get him to the toilet before he's soiled himself. Some parents are even able to prompt their child to eliminate by using a particular cue, such as a whispered "pssst."

The benefits of elimination communication include no diaper rashes or smelly diaper pails, fewer diapers used (which saves money and contributes to a healthier environment), as well as not having to train an obstinate two- or three-year-old later. People who have used the method also say it strengthens the bond between parent and child as it requires a great deal of closeness and natural communication.

So, is this method effective? It can be, for the parent who's truly diligent in following it. Experts say it's more about training the parents than the children. Infants are really too immature to understand that they need to signal you when they're ready to go, although they may learn to relax their bowels in response to your cue. Mostly, it's a matter of the parent learning to read babies' signs that a bowel movement is imminent. Of course, this requires a huge time commitment. You have to be constantly in your children's close proximity in order to know when they're ready. And often there are false alarms, so you may be running your children to the toilet quite often only to find that no tinkle is forthcoming. On the other hand, there will be times that you'll miss the cue, in which case you'll be doing a lot of upholstery scrubbing. This method is also very impractical when you're out in public. If you think one of your twins is ready to poop, will you be able to make it to the store bathroom in time? And who wants to expose their infants to the germs of a public restroom anyway? And what if there's an embarrassing accident in the middle of Macy's? Some parents compensate for these factors by using a combination of elimination communication (at home) and traditional diapering (in public).

With these benefits and drawbacks in mind, is it possible to use this method if you have multiples? Well, technically it's possible—anything's possible!—but is this really how you want to spend your life with your twins? It seems like a lot of time that could be spent on other things during your babies' precious first year of life. And this method also makes it much more difficult to leave the twins with others to give you a much-needed break! Of course, if you work outside the home or don't have enough time within the home to closely monitor your child (because you work from home or have other children to attend to), this method will fail. If you think you're up to trying it with your twins, then go for it! You have nothing to lose (except maybe your newly uphol-stered couch). My prediction, though, is that this potty training trend won't become the norm—especially among parents of multiples!

Points to Ponder

What do you think . . . is it possible to potty train infants? Would it be more challenging for the parents of twins?

Have you tried elimination communication or would you be willing to? Why or why not?

Do you think that elimination communication will be the preferred method of toilet training in the future, or is it just a fad?

Polar body twinning occurs when an unfertilized egg splits in two, and then each divided piece is fertilized by sperm from a different male. The resulting children have genes from the same mother, but different fathers. Because the father's DNA determines the sex of a child, polar body twins can be either boy/girl twins or same sex twins.

Older Children: Dealing with Jealousy

If you have an older child—or two or three (bless you!)—you may find that they don't consider your twins quite as adorable as everyone else does. They might become jealous of all the attention their little siblings get from others, or they may resent that you have less time to spend with them because you're dealing with the babies. This is natural, but there are ways to discourage this kind of resentment. It's important to be proactive and nip it in the bud before it gets to be a real problem. Tara Coleran, mother of Brett, almost three, and one-year-old identical twins, Brady and Aidan, told me, "Our children are twenty-one months apart. I believe now that they will be great friends as they grow up, but it didn't all start that way! It's hard for a toddler to adjust to having two new siblings, but my husband and I have done our best at making it easy for him. We try to take time out of the day to spend with just our oldest, even if it is for only ten minutes. It means the world to him! I can't say that I've dealt with the sibling rivalry end of things yet since they are still so young, but I have dealt with jealousy. We just make sure now that Brett has his special time with us each day."

Twins Tips

HELPING OLDER CHILDREN ADJUST TO THEIR TWIN SIBLINGS

- Avoid making your older child the "nanny." If she's constantly being called on to take care of the twins, she'll resent the extra work that's been created for her with the twins' birth. Instead, encourage her to interact with your twins in positive activities together, like singing songs or going for walks.

- Respect your older child's right to privacy. He shouldn't have to share everything with the twins. Allow him to have things that are just for him, and enforce rules limiting your twins' time in his room. Nothing makes an older sibling angrier than having little brothers or sisters in their "stuff"!

- If strangers are giving your twins all of the attention, remind them of how special your older child is, too! Tell people how great your older child is doing in school or what a great artist she is! Let her hear that you're proud of her.

- Help your older child understand that the twins are his, too. Avoid calling the twins "mommy's babies," and emphasize that he's getting new sisters! They are a gift to him, as well as to you. Try to promote family unity, of which your older child is still a very important part.

- Give your older child some one-on-one time. I know this is difficult when the twins are young, but it's very important. Perhaps Daddy can take the older child on a father/son trip to McDonald's or to play miniature golf. Emphasize to your older child that this is his very own special time with Daddy or Mommy. Perhaps the grandparents can also be enlisted to make sure that your older child continues to get individual attention.

Points to Ponder

If you have an older child (or more), how did she react when the twins were first born? Was she happy, jealous—or a little of both?

Does your older child ever resent that the twins get lots of attention from others? In what ways have you made him feel special, too?

Do you find that you have less time to devote to your older child(ren)? In what ways can you and your partner plan to give all of your children equal time?

When Twins Are Affected by TTTS

Twin to Twin Transfusion Syndrome (TTTS) is a condition that can affect identical twins who share a common placenta during pregnancy. With this condition, the placenta may be shared unequally between the twins, leaving one baby with too small a share of the placenta to receive the necessary nutrients to develop normally. This baby will also suffer from little to no amniotic fluid. The other twin may become overloaded with blood, which puts a strain on this baby's heart to the point that it may develop heart failure. This baby may also develop too much amniotic fluid. There is a 1 in 930 chance of having TTTS in pregnancy. Before TTTS could be diagnosed by ultrasound, less than 10 percent of twins with the condition survived. Now the odds of survival have greatly improved, thanks to medical intervention during pregnancy and after birth. Because the consequences and outcomes of TTTS are so diverse, this book cannot begin to address this subject adequately. Many parents of TTTS twins (as well as those parents who have lost twins from this condition) have told me that they've benefited greatly from support groups. One such organization is the Twin to Twin Transfusion Syndrome Foundation. You can visit them on the Web at www.tttsfoundation.org.

Kristy Fitzgerald's identical twin boys, Anthony and Alex, are TTTS survivors. Born on December 21, 2003, ten weeks early, they had a "rough first year," as Kristy characterizes it. As a result of being the recipient of TTTS, Anthony has cerebral palsy, but Kristy is thrilled that he took his first three steps at the age of two-and-a-half! Following is a poem that Kristy wrote after her twins were born. She recommends that all parents write a "birth poem" to their twins that they can read when they get older.

Twins Tale

FROM GOD'S HANDS
Kristy Fitzgerald

I'm alone, numb, so scared. I'm shaking inside.
They say you're here. I can't hear you.
The pumps of the airbag sound loud, resuscitation . . .
Oh, God, Twin A is out.

Now they try for you, little B. So many people around,
but do you know I'm here? I hear a faint cry.
They're working on you. Daddy's here now.
A quick glimpse and now you're gone.
Six hours later, I'm still awake.
I want to see you and feel you, but they won't let me go.
Try and rest they say. I can't. You need my milk.
That's all I can do for you.

Daddy goes alone. He's so sad, I think he cried.
He's not himself. I'm scared. He can't go again, he says.

Finally, my turn. You're 10 hours old.
Twin A, 2 pounds, 10 ounces, 15 inches long,
you're so small, you're red, you're puffy.
Mama loves you, Alex, but the nurse is confused.
They thought the big one was Anthony. This is the big one?

They take me to B, the little one.
Oh, God, 2 pounds, 1 ounce, 13 inches long,
too small, you're too small. You are gray, bony, and so still.
Don't cry. STOP crying. Be strong. Breathe, pray, breathe.
I feel faint, I need to sit.

Are they breathing? What's this? What's that? It's so loud, unnatural.
I HATE my body. You let me down.
God, don't take them, please, please give them strength.

Anthony is A. Call him Anthony. Alex is B. That's his name, please.
Write it. I want you to call them by name.
I have to leave today. Sydney needs me, too.
I'll be back tomorrow and every day.

One week later, I can hold you now. You feel warm,
but frail. I may break you. You sleep most of the time.
Rest, grow, please come home.

Seven more weeks, no more apnea, no more oxygen,
no more machines. I'm so excited.
Anthony is ready. What a big boy, 5 pounds!
But wait, what about brother? Oh no, you'll be alone.
I'm sorry, Alex.
We don't want to leave you.

Three days later. He's ready? I don't believe it.
I need to hear the doctors say it.
"Do you want us to potty train him?" they ask. I laugh.
I can't stop smiling. Little Alex the Great, 4 1/2 pounds now!

What a beautiful day. I am soooo happy.
I feel as if you were just born.
It's our beginning. You're both finally home.
Finally, I get to know you.
I want to hold you every second. I need to kiss you,
smell you, love you, and watch you.
Thank you, thank you, thank you, God. I am grateful!

Points to Ponder

Did your twins develop TTTS or some other medical condition? How has this affected them and your family?

Were your twins premature? How did this affect their health and long-term development?

How can you find support and help for your family if your child has a disability?

Have you or your partner considered writing a poem or a letter to your twins about how you felt when they were born? What feelings would you like to express?

Coping with a Disability

Parents of multiples are already overwhelmed with the extra care required of more than one baby, but when one or both children are disabled, the challenges can become particularly acute. Multiples do have a slightly higher chance of having a physical or mental impairment because of various factors more common to multiple births, such as TTTS and premature birth. Thus, parents must be extra-vigilant about reducing the stress in their lives, developing a bond with their twins, and paying special attention to the needs of older siblings who may feel neglected when your time and attention is naturally focused on your youngest children. If one twin comes home from the hospital sooner than the other, a bond may form more quickly with the child who is home. Conversely, the child with special needs may naturally be the recipient of more attention, thus depriving parents of the time needed to form a bond with the other twin. Thus, it's important to be sure that the emotional and physical needs of all of your children are being met—not an easy task when you're exhausted and stressed. It is particularly important during this time to willingly accept any help available. Don't hesitate to ask for assistance, even if it's just to have someone sit with your children for a half-hour while you take a much-needed break. And ask your doctor to recommend any organizations or agencies that might provide you with information or help.

Terri Mobbs, mother of identical twin boys, one of whom has cerebral palsy, has some advice to share with parents who have a disabled child. Following that is a poem written by John C. Flewellen, father of twin boys with Crohn's disease.

Twins Tips

HOW FAMILIES CAN DEAL WITH
ONE TWIN HAVING DELAYS OR PROBLEMS
Terri Mobbs

- Enjoy their bond as twins, but also treat them as two separate, individual children with different interests and needs.

- Find a support group online or in your area.

- Acknowledge each twin's strengths and differences, but do not expect them to be at equal places.

- Communicate physical abilities or limitations to other children and others around you.

- Keep your marriage a priority and work together.

- Spend time individually with each child doing what he or she wants to do.

- Be prepared for opposition to keeping the twins together in educational settings.

- Take time to grieve the loss of your dreams, but do not stay in a grieving state.

- Develop standard responses to the questions you receive in public about your twins (Are they twins? Then why isn't he walking? What is wrong with him? etc.).

- Get information and medical services that are available for children with special needs.

Twins Tale

WHY, LORD, WHY?
John C. Flewellen

Sitting at my desk,
With a tear in my eye,
Asking the old question,
Why, Lord, why?

Why my twin boys
Have to have Crohn's?
My heart breaks every time
I hear their moans.

I wish I could take it,
Take their pain away.
But for now
I can only pray.

I pray for the healing in their bodies,
I pray for solid minds,
I pray they keep their heads up,
And cherish YOU all the time.

Someday, I know,
A cure will be found
And when that day comes
A smile will replace the frown.

Points to Ponder

Is one or both of your twins developmentally delayed? What are the circumstances?

In what ways does having a disabled child affect your family dynamics?

What types of assistance or activities help you deal with the challenges associated with caring for a disabled child and meeting the needs of all family members?

Twins Trivia
WHAT IS VANISHING TWIN SYNDROME?

Because the diagnosis of twins is happening earlier in pregnancy, thanks to the use of ultrasound, doctors are discovering more cases of Vanishing Twin Syndrome (VTS). This occurs when twins are initially conceived, but one mysteriously disappears during pregnancy, resulting in a singleton pregnancy. In other words, one twin is miscarried; the other survives. The miscarried twin's fetal tissue is usually absorbed by the mother, the placenta, or the other twin. This condition most often occurs in the first trimester, so many VTS cases go undetected if an ultrasound is not performed in the first three months of pregnancy. Some estimates say that one in eight people may have started as a twin, but only one in seventy pregnancies actually results in a twin birth. VTS usually poses no physical problems for the mother or surviving child, but there is often an emotional component whereby parents grieve over losing a child but are relieved that one has survived.

Twins Tips
BE ON THE LOOKOUT FOR HAIR TOURNIQUETS

I clearly remember the day I thought that one of my boys would lose a toe! The twins were about six weeks old, and my mother-in-law was visiting from Alaska. She was bathing Caleb in the sink when she noticed that one of his toes was turning blue! Upon closer examination, we realized that a piece of hair had become wound around two of his toes so tightly that it was cutting off the circulation. In fact, the strand was embedded so deeply that we could only see the cut lines in his toes and the hair stretched between the two toes. Holding Caleb carefully so that he wouldn't wiggle, we managed to slice the hair between his toes with a small knife and slowly unwind it. It was difficult to know if we had retrieved all of the hair, but fortunately the blood began flowing back into the toes and the blue color disappeared. I was so grateful to my mother-in-law for noticing the problem because it could have resulted in the loss of one or two toes! Even though I had already successfully steered two other children through infancy, I had never heard of this phenomenon or been warned of the possibility.

Experts call this a "hair tourniquet," and it can be a real threat to infants. Hair can get wrapped around fingers and toes—and even penises! (In fact, I read an article where a baby girl lost her clitoris due to "hair tourniquet syndrome.") Even pet hair or loose threads from a blanket or piece of clothing can become entangled. Because human hair is so thin and tends to contract when it dries, you may not even notice a problem until the appendage begins to show signs of distress. With multiples, it might be easier to overlook a hair because we tend to get into "assembly line mode" when bathing or dressing our children and may not be as observant. Serious sleep deprivation may also play a factor in missing the signs of a hair tourniquet! So, be extra vigilant. (Who doesn't love to check out those adorable little fingers and toes anyway?) If your babies wear mittens or gloves, check their fingers for signs of wrapped threads once they're removed. Check toes after removing booties or slippers. If a child is inconsolable and you can't figure out why, consider that he could be in pain from a hair tourniquet.

If you find a problem, you'll need a sharp tool like a small knife to cut the hair if you don't see a loose end. Get some help to hold your child still while you remove the hair so no one gets hurt. If you're unable to disentangle the hair or thread, contact your physician immediately. He may recommend soaking the limb in a hair-dissolving solution (like Nair), or have you bring the baby into the office or emergency room. (If you can't reach a doctor, head to the hospital or urgent care center right away.) It's important not to delay removing the hair because serious infection or limb/digit loss can occur.

I have long hair, so there's always lots of my "shedding" around the house, but remember that all women tend to lose a lot of hair soon after giving birth due to hormonal changes—regardless of length. This can make the possibility of hair tourniquets more likely. So, frequently examine those little fingers, toes, and private parts!

Points to Ponder

Do you ever find yourself shifting into "assembly line mode" when you're washing, feeding, or dressing your babies? How can you slow down and appreciate their sweet smell and perfection?

Have you ever had a scary moment with your twins, such as discovering a hair tourniquet, having one of them fall, or an illness? How did you handle it?

Long-Distance Travel with Infant Twins

If the thought of hopping on a plane with your baby twins sounds daunting, you're not alone! My twins are now two-and-a-half years old, and I still haven't taken them on more than a two-hour car trip to their grandparents' house! (And Caleb got carsick and puked all over the car only twenty minutes into one of those trips, so I'm still not feeling very eager to travel!) But other parents are much braver than I and have successfully taken their infant twins across the country . . . and even across the world! Twins mom Deanne Whiteley has taken her twins on countless coast-to-coast flights across the United States, as well as twice to Australia (once, believe it or not, without her husband). Deanne has my nomination for bravest mother on the planet! Needless to say, if you're very organized and well prepared, you can accomplish your travel plans with your sanity intact. So, I'll turn the reins over to Deanne, a true travel expert, and let her tell you about one of her trips and offer some excellent advice if you're contemplating your own long-distance trip with your twin babies.

Twins Tale

TWIN TIME WARP
Deanne Whiteley

In the early hours of a crisp, clear fall morning, we piled our luggage high on the sidewalk outside our house. The cab driver looked at us in dismay when he spied the three giant suitcases, two backpacks, diaper bag, travel documents satchel, two car seats, and a double jog stroller.

"Yikes!" he said. "You forgot the kitchen sink! Where on earth are you going?"

"To the opposite end," I laughed.

"Australia," my husband Chris interceded.

I moved my twelve-month-old son from one hip to the other. The cab driver opened the trunk and sighed loudly as he attempted to squeeze our belongings into the dusty compartment—a seemingly impossible task. Chris handed me the other baby and began fitting the car seats in the back of the cab. Juggling a twin on each hip, I wondered just how long this day would be. Amazingly, everything fit in the cab, and we headed off for Logan Airport with luggage squeezed around our knees.

The rest of the morning proceeded as planned. Our luggage was checked, seats and tickets allocated. We were then herded along with other anxious business and pleasure travelers to the back of the security line, which appeared to snake halfway around the airport. There's something about airport security that is reminiscent of a fraternity hazing as you take off half your clothing, empty your pockets, and remove your watch and anything else that might set off the machine. Hurriedly, you do all this under the watchful eye of an overbearing security attendant and a crowd of onlookers. Of course, as a parent, it's even worse because you then must pull your sleeping kids out of the stroller, unbundle the babies, orderly sort your belongings into standard gray boxes, and load the rest of your carry-ons through the screening machine. Oh, and while balancing two babies, you must also collapse the stroller and attempt to push it through an opening in the screening machine, which is obviously no match for a giant jog stroller. Now the line behind you is even longer and you're sweating buckets. Eventually, the attendant is convinced that you're no threat, and you now have the pleasure of lugging the stroller off the conveyor belt. You reassemble it and wheel over to a woman frantically waving something that resembles a magic wand. Of course, nothing is found but stale Cheerios. You get the "all clear" nod, gather your family and belongings, and then reassemble, redress, repack, and move on from this obligatory stop. On this day, the whole process took nearly an hour.

Hot and sweaty from lugging the car seats and carry-ons, and maneuvering a stroller around meandering travelers, we arrived at our gate. Apparently on this domestic airline, early boarding for families was a thing of the past, so we joined the massive line of lingering passengers and waited to be ushered onto the plane. Finally, the four of us—twelve-month-old twins Bailey and Zander, Chris, and I—boarded the first of two flights on our transpacific journey.

We struggled down the narrow aisle with babes on hips, bags on shoulders, and a car seat dragging behind us. Of course, we were seated all the way at the back of the plane. By the time we reached our seats, I was completely soaked in sweat. Chris stored our luggage while I strapped in the car seats and secured the babies. Just as I plopped down in my seat, an oversized man plastered with sweat and a comb-over that started below his ear alleged that I was sitting in his seat. With a sigh I pulled out our tickets to show him that, in fact, these were our seats. As I flipped through the tickets, I discovered to my horror that of the four seats we occupied, only baby Zander was sitting in the correct seat! It appeared that all four of us were seated at opposite ends of the plane—even the twins were ticketed to sit by themselves!

"Didn't you check the tickets at the reservation desk?" I whispered frantically to Chris as I wiped sweat from my forehead.

"No, I thought you checked the tickets. Besides, what kind of moron would seat babies by themselves?" replied Chris.

"No idea. Personally, I'd be happy to have some baby-free time, but I can't imagine that anyone else would be satisfied with this arrange-ment," I said sarcastically.

I turned to the man who was now tapping on my seat, forced a smile, and attempted to explain our predicament. He listened, which I took to be a good sign. Wrong. After I finished my exposé, he said, "So, ya gonna move then?"

Well, that was pretty clear. Chris unbuckled the car seats while I tried to flag down an air steward. Ah, got one. Once again, I began to explain our seating drama. I found that as I talked, I continually had to duck as passengers precariously forced luggage into the storage compartment above my head. I wasn't even sure the steward was really listening; he seemed preoccupied with shuffling bags around and closing the com-partment doors. When I eventually finished my account of events, the steward just shrugged his shoulders and said, "Well, either you go to your assigned seats or you wait until the passengers sitting next to your seats have boarded and ask if they'd be willing to swap."

It didn't sound like a great plan—or even a plan at all. But, as there didn't seem to be anything else to do, I watched and waited. As passen-gers began taking their seats in rows around us, I approached several of the sympathetic looking ones, and with my brightest smile, asked if they'd be willing to help us out. To my relief, someone finally agreed.

Okay, now we had two seats together, so we just needed to find one or possibly two more cooperative passengers.

I marched up the aisle to Bailey's seat and quickly explained to the passenger seated in the middle of the row that he would shortly be accompanied by a screaming one-year-old. However, I'd be happy to trade seats with him if he didn't mind moving a few rows down. That did the trick. Finally, we had two seats: an aisle and a middle seat. I put the baby in the aisle seat, thinking that would be nicer for my window companion. Just as I tightened the last buckle on my son, the air steward informed me that infants in car seats must be seated next to the window.

The current window-seat occupant clearly did not want to move. She sat tight-lipped looking out the window as if to say, "No, I'm not even going to engage in any kind of conversation with you." I turned to the steward, whose only advice was to move quickly because apparently I was now delaying our departure. This was surely too unbelievable to be true. Not certain what to do, I chased the steward down the aisle and explained that my window companion had refused to move. Perhaps if he asked, the result might be different. The air steward agreed to help, and within minutes we were all buckled into our new seats. I apologized to the passenger who had just been made to move, but she simply turned her head in the opposite direction and put on an eye mask and headphones.

I took a deep breath. Finally, we could settle in and prepare for the next six hours. I was exhausted already, and we hadn't even left the ground! As the plane was taxiing down the runway, I realized that Chris had the diaper bag at the back of the plane. I had planned on giving the baby a bottle of milk on takeoff to help equalize his little ears. *Oh, well, I thought, I guess I'll just see how things go.* As the plane began its ascent, it was clear by the expression on my fellow passenger's face that things were not going so well. Baby Bailey was crying, his mouth was opening wider with each intake of air, and his volume was increasing rapidly. He'd probably hit crescendo shortly. I turned around in my seat and waved to Chris, but he wasn't looking. I yelled out his name, but my voice was drowned out by the drum of the engines. The seatbelt sign was still on, and the plane remained on a steep incline. I noticed a scrap of paper sticking out of the seat pocket. I grabbed it and scrawled in pink crayon, "Please pass to the guy with a Red Sox cap and baby at the back of the plane. Chris, send up milk for your son." I passed it to the lady seated behind me. And so, in something reminiscent of grade school, the note traveled all the way down to the back of the plane, passing through hand after hand. Just as Bailey was hitting crescendo forte, I saw a bottle sailing up the aisle, seat over seat, hand-to-hand, until it finally reached its destination: my son's hungry little mouth. *Wawawawaaaaaaa! Ahhhhhhh . . . Suck. Suck. Suck.* Silence.

After six hours, we finally landed in Los Angeles. We collected our bags and headed to the airport hotel where we'd try to get some rest for the next seven hours. Due to the east/west coast time difference, there's often a fairly long layover between domestic and international flights. We would have a ten-hour layover before our international flight departed. We all took a long nap. It was good to lie flat on our backs and enjoy a nice meal and a much-needed glass of wine. All too quickly the day had passed, the sun had set, and we limbo travelers packed up our belongings (sippy cups, bottles, wipes, diapers, toys, soiled clothes, baby food, car seats, and so forth) and headed out to the hotel foyer to catch the airport shuttle back to LAX International Airport. Once again, we lined up for our tickets (this time checking our seating arrangements), struggled back through security, and finally, after what felt like a marathon effort, made it to our gate at 11 P.M.

Traveling to Australia is like entering a time warp. You leave East Coast America and fly six hours to her West Coast. You arrive on the West Coast with a bonus three hours added to your day. You leave the West Coast (usually Los Angeles) on a midnight flight, and after fifteen hours of flying you arrive in Australia in the early morning two days after you left. Confused? Essentially, when you cross the international date line, a whole day simply disappears, just like that. There's not even a satisfying puff of smoke. It's not all bad news, though. Should you brave a return trip from Australia to America, you will actually arrive on the West Coast of America about the same time you left Australia, if not a few minutes before your flight departed 9,000 miles earlier.

As we pre-boarded our transpacific flight, we were greeted by the captain and his crew. They welcomed us on the plane with beautiful New Zealand accents, and when they saw our arms laden with babies, car seats, and bags, they enthusiastically offered assistance, removing items from our arms as we passed by. They helped us store our luggage and get settled. They held our twins and happily cooed over them. Within minutes, we knew each staff member by name, and they knew ours and our children's names. We were seated comfortably at the bulkhead, all together in our seats with belts fastened ready for takeoff. The experience was blissful. We sat there and smiled at each other, watching the hubbub of activity as other passengers stored their luggage and located their seats.

Sitting in the bulkhead on a Boeing 747 has the added advantage of extra leg room and pull-down bassinets. There isn't really a disadvantage to these seats other than the location of a giant video screen in front of your face. *I hope we like the movie,* I thought. *It would be rather hard not to watch it.* I felt like I was sitting in the front row at the cinema. Even though we were all seated together, we had decided to each be responsible for one baby. So when our baby slept, we could also sleep. This time, I decided to take my chances with baby Zander. We read a few stories, and then dinner was served: beef Wellington with seasonal vegetables and a nice glass of red wine. This was all rather civilized considering our prior flight, during which we had all survived on a mini packet of pretzels that would leave even a supermodel famished.

The movie screen sprang to life, flashing colors and shapes before my son's eyes. Unfortunately, this was more stimulating than relaxing. As I tried to soothe Zander to sleep, I watched the opening scene of the movie sans sound. Renee Zellweger was running around with a large butt squeezed into a tight mini skirt. Then she was jumping from a plane into a pigsty. Ahh, it must be *Bridget Jones's Diary*! Maybe I'd watch a bit of the movie once Zander fell asleep. Surely, it couldn't be much longer; this little baby was so tired. Half an hour later, I was still pacing up and down the plane with an overtired baby who just couldn't fall asleep. I'd already dosed him up with Benadryl, but that had simply made him more agitated. I was sure that if I could just get him to relax, he'd fall asleep. *He must be exhausted,* I told myself. *After all, it is 4 A.M. East Coast time!* Heck, I was tired. I'd have happily closed my eyes and drifted off to sleep, especially if someone were gently rocking me.

An hour into the movie, Zander was close to hysterical, and I had pretty much run out of ideas. I'd long given up attempting to get him to sleep. I was just frantically focused on trying to calm him down before my fellow passengers opened the emergency exit and pushed us out mid-flight. It was probably from an hour's worth of crying, I reasoned, but this little baby felt incredibly hot to me. Not knowing what else to do and needing to feel like I was doing something to help this impossible situation, I decided to take his temperature. Maybe he had a fever, an earache, a tummy ache, a hair wrapped tightly around his toe—who knew? I hoped the number on a thermometer would give me a clue as to this little baby's frantic state. I placed him in the pull-down bassinet, removed his pajamas and diaper, and then with expert efficiency inserted a rectal thermometer. No sooner had I done this than a stream of pee shot up into my face. Stunned, I closed my mouth and immediately moved my head as I frantically searched for something to cover this exploding fountain. Incredibly, the stream continued to shoot directly up onto the movie screen and across Hugh Grant's face! Quickly, I stifled the flow with a clean diaper and began wiping the screen with a moist baby wipe. As I wiped Hugh down, I turned to look at my husband, seeking moral support. Instead, I saw my husband and son Bailey sleeping soundly with their eyes shut tight. To my horror, I also noticed several stunned passengers with mouths agape. I overheard one woman say, "I can't believe she let her baby pee on the movie screen!" I turned away and hung my head in embarrassment, bundled up the baby and headed for the only private place I could think of: the lavatory. I sat in that cramped, brightly lit box for at least twenty minutes, too embarrassed and exhausted to return to my seat.

Sometime later, I realized I was still holding the thermometer in my hand. It turns out that Zander did have a slight fever, so after giving him some medicine, I eventually managed to calm him down. By the end of the movie, he was finally closing his heavy, little eyelids, and we both fell into a deep slumber for several hours.

I can't express the relief I felt when the plane finally touched down on solid ground. We'd actually made it. I was home for three fabulous weeks: two weddings and a christening, and the exciting event of finally introducing our twins to their grandparents, aunties, uncles, great this and that, and extended family and friends. However, first and foremost, I needed a shower and some rest. Even though I'd showered the morning we left Boston, bizarrely that was now three days ago.

I shuddered as I thought about the return trip. I wondered if there were another way—I could really use a time-travel machine!

Twins Tips

HELPFUL HINTS FOR PARENTS TRAVELING WITH MULTIPLES
Deanne Whiteley

Is there any need to call the airline prior to our departure?

Even though these days you no longer need to confirm airline reservations, I highly recommend calling the airline you'll be traveling on and confirming the following:

- Flight details, dates, departure times, and the recommended time you should be at the airport (then add an extra thirty minutes). Everything takes longer when you have little ones, and the unexpected always happens.

- Confirm your seats and ensure you are all seated together. On smaller planes where the seats are either two or three seats to a row, request rows immediately behind or opposite each other, so both parents can help out during the flight. This arrangement will also make it easier to share a diaper bag.

- I always request the bulkhead on international flights, but it's typically given on a first-come, first-served basis, with preference given to infants twelve months and under.

Should we purchase tickets for our little ones?

It always seemed like a waste of money to buy seats for our twins when they were young enough to be lap children (under two years)—that is, until we actually flew five hours with two squirming babies on our laps.

- For children under two years, you have three options: use your lap child pass and hope there are spare seats near you on the flight; buy one seat for both babies to share or switch in and out of; or, the most expensive option, buy seats for both children.

- It's a personal decision whether you choose to have lap babies or buy seats at a slightly discounted child rate. However, when making this decision, consider the length of your flight, layovers, season (if it's peak travel time, there probably won't be any spare seats), and total travel time to your destination.

We bought airplane seats for our twins. Should we take their car seats on the plane or check them?

Somehow, the plane seatbelt didn't seem to hold our babies in their seats. When our twins were younger, they simply slipped out, and when they were older they quickly learned how to flip the buckle and escape out into the aisle.

- Despite the cumbersome task of lugging car seats around the airport, we have always found it worthwhile at the end of a long flight. Our twins are more manageable and sleep longer when seated in a car seat. On short trips where we didn't use the car seats, we spent the entire time juggling squirmy babies. (But, depending on your tolerance level, sometimes it's worth saving the extra money!)

- If you plan on using car seats on the plane, make sure the airline doesn't have any restrictions on their use. Some airlines require pre-authorization for car seats from their head office, which can take one to two weeks.

Should I pack snacks, milk/formula, and food for the flight?

A flight attendant once offered me a box of fifty creamers and suggested I pour them into a bottle! The flight would have been on the ground again before I finished.

- If your twins are drinking milk (not formula), find out if the airline carries any cow's milk on board. Many airlines only offer small creamers.

- Most supermarkets sell small boxes of UHT milk, which don't need to be refrigerated until opened.

- If you have purchased seats for your children, make sure you request an age-appropriate meal (especially on an international flight). In my experience, meals usually come in adult (regular, vegetarian, diabetic), child/toddler, and infant.

- All planes have hot water on board, and attendants can wash bottles and sippy cups for you. They also have bottled water that can be used for powdered formula.

- Bring enough formula for your entire travel time and a little extra for emergencies. Also bring jarred baby food or, if your little ones are beyond that, lots of snacks. I often pack a small, soft cool pack with extra drinks and my twins' favorite snacks.

Besides food, what else should I pack in the diaper bag for the flight and transit time?

What and how much you pack will depend on the age of your children and the length of your flight. I'm typically an over-packer and take more than we probably need, but I take comfort in knowing that we'll be prepared if stranded in an airport. I frequently pack two diaper bags in case we're not seated together. You can also split your bags and put diapers, wipes, clothing, and a medical kit in one, and formula, snacks, drinks, and toys in the other. Here's what I pack:

- Enough diapers, wipes, and diaper rash cream for the entire travel time (flight and transit time) and two to four extras for emergencies.

- At least one spare outfit per child and an extra shirt for yourself and partner. (No matter how careful you are, accidents happen regularly with little ones.) Onesies are great for infants as they are small and don't take up much space. For long-haul flights, you may want extra outfits and pajamas or a footed play/sleep suit.

- Bottles or sippy cups. Bottles with disposable liners save on cleaning up; you can even bring extra nipples and dump the used ones in a Ziploc bag.

- If your little ones use pacifiers, bring them (and some extra ones). Sucking is very soothing and can also help equalize ear pressure. Alternatively, try having your children suck on a bottle, drink from a sippy cup, eat/suck on snacks, or nurse.

- Be sure to pack an emergency medicine kit, complete with pain relief medicine, thermometer, and anything else you think you might need. Benadryl can make children sleepy; it can also have the opposite effect. If you are thinking about using this medicine, be sure to check with your pediatrician first and do a trial a few days before you fly. (The last thing you want is a hyperactive child.)

Can I nurse comfortably on the flight?

I have expressed milk on many flights. Due to our seating arrangements (usually baby in car seat in the middle seat and I by the window), I'm sure my fellow passengers were none the wiser.

- If you plan on nursing or pumping, consider requesting a window seat for yourself. For added privacy, tie a sarong between your seat and the seat in front of you.

- Many airports have discreet family rooms that you can use upon request.

How can I keep my children entertained?

Surprisingly, gift wrapping small, inexpensive new toys or toys my twins haven't played with in a while has yielded just as much delight as giving an expensive new toy. Half the excitement is in opening the present, which can take some time for little hands if you wrap it well.

- Bring your children's favorite (age-appropriate) toys and loveys.

- My twins' occupational therapist suggested that for long flights, it is helpful to offer children different stimuli (for example, soft, hard, rough, smooth, stacking, shaking, etc.). She suggested colored sand in a tightly sealed clear plastic bottle, shakers, and small, plastic containers that little hands can unscrew or pull the lids off, filled with play dough, ribbons, crayons, or toys (whatever is appropriate for your children).

- If you are comfortable with your children watching TV, consider using a laptop or small DVD player to show age-appropriate shows such as *Sesame Street, Baby Einstein,* and *Thomas the Tank Engine.* Invest in an extended battery and voltage adapter if you are traveling overseas.

Should I take my double stroller or buy umbrella strollers? What about backpacks?

If you take your expensive double stroller to the gate, I recommend placing it in a heavy-duty bag to prevent scratches, tears, and other damage.

- Umbrella strollers are light and can be stored in the overhead compartment on most airplanes. You can also buy connectors to join the two strollers together.

- A jog stroller can be useful at your final destination, but its biggest advantage is that it is able to carry more of your stuff without tipping. In the past, we have been able to strap the twins' car seats to the back of the stroller, leaving us to carry just the diaper bag.

- Another creative option is to carry your children in backpacks or have one child in a stroller and one in a backpack.

- You can buy special carry bags for car seats that make them easier to lug around an airport.

- If you are a frequent traveler, consider investing in a car seat that converts to a stroller. Many online and baby catalogs sell these clever seats.

Additional tips:

- Consider booking a room in an airport hotel if you have a long layover between flights (six hours or more), and be sure to request a day rate. You'll all get on your next flight refreshed and ready for the next adventure.

- Many taxi companies have a minivan service that can be booked up to a week in advance. There is usually a $5–10 service charge on top of the regular fee, and you can arrange to have them pick you up upon your return. (Beats waiting in the taxi line.)

Points to Ponder

Have you taken your first long-distance trip with your twins yet? If yes, how did it go? If no, what's stopping you?

If you have traveled with your twins, what tips do you have for making the trip more manageable for everyone?

What funny or horrible stories do you have about traveling with your twins, whether they be shorter car trips or longer plane trips?

Intriguing Twins
ALICE AND NELLIE CLARKE

Imagine having twins in the year 1900. No ultrasound machines. No apnea monitors. No neonatal intensive care units. No modern medical equipment of any kind. In fact, you may not even have known you were pregnant with twins! You wouldn't know to be careful about premature labor. You wouldn't have four names picked out (two boys, two girls). In fact, the odds of delivering healthy twins would have been much lower than they are today. So, it was quite a miracle when identical twins Alice and Nellie Clarke were born on June 15, 1900, in Hale, Cheshire, England.

The twins were born twenty-five minutes apart to William Clarke, a well-to-do wholesaler, and his wife Adelaide. The family never lacked for money, and the girls traveled the world with their parents, even visiting Egypt, which was quite a feat in those days. The young debutantes were quite advanced for their time in other ways, too. In an era when women rarely drove, the two women learned to drive a car. They also took over the operation of a dress shop owned by their father in Timperley, Altrincham. During World War II, they were volunteer ambulance drivers! Alice continued to drive until she was in her nineties, at which time she received her first speeding ticket—at the age of ninety-one.

The girls obviously shared a very special bond. They never married, and they claimed that they never spent more than a half-hour apart all their lives. They lived independently until they moved into a nursing home in 1995.

On June 15, 2000, the twins celebrated their 100th birthdays by hosting a garden party featuring strawberries and cream and a New Orleans-style jazz band. Their most memorable gift was a telegram from Queen Elizabeth II congratulating them on their milestone birthdays.

Nellie died on April 12, 2001, just two months shy of her 101st birthday. Her sister followed five months later, on September 16. These amazing twins hold the distinction of being Britain's most long-lived twins. When asked the secret to their longevity, the twins advised people to always behave properly and to be happy.

Despite the odds, Alice and Nellie Clarke lived long and full lives. Thanks to modern medicine, we'll soon be seeing more and more twins living to the ripe old age of one hundred! Hopefully, their lives will be as full and blessed as those of Alice and Nellie.

Twins Trivia

MOST POPULAR NAMES OF TWINS BORN IN 2005
ACCORDING TO THE SOCIAL SECURITY ADMINISTRATION

1. Jacob, Joshua
2. Matthew, Michael
3. Daniel, David
4. Faith, Hope
5. Ethan, Evan
6. Taylor, Tyler
7. Isaac, Isaiah
8. Joseph, Joshua
9. Nathan, Nicholas
10. Madison, Mason
11. Hailey, Hannah
12. Madison, Morgan
13. Alexander, Andrew
14. Elijah, Isaiah
15. Jordan, Justin
16. Mackenzie, Madison
17. Alexander, Nicholas
18. Caleb, Joshua
19. Emma, Ethan
20. Jonathan, Joshua
21. Emily, Ethan
22. Alexander, Benjamin
23. Andrew, Matthew
24. Benjamin, Samuel
25. James, John
26. Matthew, Nicholas
27. Brandon, Brian
28. Ella, Emma
29. Alexander, Zachary
30. Dylan, Tyler
31. Hannah, Sarah
32. Madison, Matthew
33. Christian, Christopher
34. Faith, Grace
35. Jacob, Jordan
36. Jacob, Matthew
37. Jaden, Jordan
38. Alexander, Anthony
39. Brandon, Bryan
40. Emily, Sarah
41. Ethan, Nathan
42. Jacob, Joseph
43. Jordan, Joshua
44. Landon, Logan
45. Olivia, Sophia
46. Ashley, Emily
47. Elizabeth, Emily
48. Elizabeth, Katherine
49. Jeremy, Joshua
50. John, Joseph
51. Nathan, Noah
52. Nicholas, Noah
53. Nicholas, Zachary
54. Alexander, Christopher
55. Christopher, Michael
56. Jacob, Zachary
57. Jason, Justin
58. Abigail, Allison
59. Amy, Emily
60. Andrew, Nicholas
61. Benjamin, William
62. Christopher, Nicholas
63. Ella, Ethan
64. Gabriella, Isabella

65. Isabella, Sophia
66. Jeremiah, Joshua
67. Megan, Morgan
68. Samuel, Sophia
69. Aidan, Ava
70. Alexander, Alexis
71. Andrew, Anthony
72. Andrew, Ethan
73. Andrew, William
74. Ava, Olivia
75. Caleb, Jacob
76. Jacob, Nicholas
77. Jacob, Ryan
78. Jake, Luke
79. Jayden, Jordan
80. John, William
81. Mark, Matthew
82. Natalie, Nathan
83. Nathaniel, Nicholas
84. Ryan, Tyler
85. Abigail, Emily
86. Anna, Emma
87. Anthony, Michael
88. Anthony, Nicholas
89. Austin, Justin
90. Benjamin, Jacob
91. Brian, Brianna
92. Christopher, Matthew
93. Daniel, Samuel
94. Gabriel, Michael
95. Haley, Hannah
96. Jada, Jaden
97. Jayden, Jaylen
98. Jonathan, Joseph
99. Kyle, Ryan
100. Logan, Lucas
101. Logan, Luke
102. Matthew, Ryan
103. Parker, Payton
104. Parker, Peyton
105. Reagan, Riley
106. Tanner, Tyler

Decoding the Mysteries of Twinship

People have always been fascinated by twins. Long ago, the Yoruba people of Nigeria would kill twins as soon as they were born (and sometimes their mother, too!) in the belief that the twins were a bad omen or that their mother had been with two men in order to conceive two babies. Fortunately, this practice is no longer carried out! The Navajo people believe that twin sons, fathered by the sun, fought off monsters using lightning bolts given to them by their father. The monsters were turned into the rock formations that are found in the western United States today. Surprisingly, many modern myths still exist about twins, such as the belief that there is always a "good twin" and a "bad twin"!

Scattered throughout this book, as you may have already discovered, are sections called Twins Trivia, which address many of the misconceptions and questions that people have about twins. In the meantime, enjoy this next story about how one mother of twins, Mary Brauer, responds to the misconceptions that her friends have about multiples.

Twins Tale

DEBUNKING THE MYTHS
Mary Brauer

Back in ancient times (yes, before televisions and even radios), twins were either reviled or revered. Due to a lack of credible facts, many people found twins very mysterious. As a result, there are still a lot of myths and skewed assumptions about them. I learned this revelation early in my pregnancy with our twins.

One day, a co-worker who is known to accurately predict the sex of an unborn baby came into my office to determine the sex of the child I was carrying. Unknown to all of us at that time, I was expecting twin boys.

As she began her examinations, she attracted a crowd of curious co-workers who gathered in my office to see her in action. Soon my tiny office filled up with people. She did all of her usual things: touched my stomach, looked at the shape of my nostrils, examined my palm and fingernails, and read the coffee grounds in the bottom of my mug. She closed her eyes for about a minute as we all waited for her pronouncement.

"I can't read it at all," she remarked. "Something definitely weird is going on in there." She turned and walked out of my office. I sat there stunned while everyone else avoided eye contact with me as they filed out of my office, whispering and huddling together. Normally, I am a very rational person, but when your hormones are surging and you're carrying a live being (or two) inside your body, you tend to get spooked a bit when a pronouncement like that is made.

When I told my non-hormonal husband about the strange experience, he chalked the whole thing up to superstition and perhaps some indigestion on my part.

Weeks later, we discovered that we were expecting twins. My co-worker looked at my stomach, shook her head and said, "You'd best prepare yourself. Twins are a whole 'nother breed!"

Wisely, I ignored her not-so-subtle warning and treated my twins as normal human babies when they arrived. However, from the get-go, I noticed that many friends and strangers asked me the oddest questions. I surveyed other parents of twins and discovered there are still a lot of myths out there about twins. So, here are some of the common ones and the true answers.

Myth: Twins skip a generation.

This is an old tale that mothers told their daughters to scare them into behaving. Many studies show that twins can occur every generation, not happen at all, or hit some misfortunate families two or three times in the same generation!

Myth: Twins have the same personality.

I don't know of any twins who share the exact likes and dislikes. Typically, each child has his or her own preferred clothes, style, and interests. However, twins are known to share similar dislikes, such as any green vegetable.

Myth: The taller/bigger twin is the first born.

Birth order doesn't have anything to do with size. Each one grows at a different rate, and many times they'll take turns being the bigger twin. Twins just do that to confuse everyone—they like to do that!

Myth: Twins have their "own language."

While it has been scientifically proven that a small percentage of twins share a private language that only they understand, most twins just gang up on their parents, caregivers, and teachers by pretending to have their own language so they can plot some sort of mayhem.

Myth: Boy/girl twins can be identical.

Unless they come up with a scientific breakthrough, it's just not possible for one egg to split and then become two different genders.

Myth: You can tell twins because they dress alike.

Most twins are hidden in society by not dressing alike and not even looking like each other.

Myth: Twins always have a built-in playmate.

At times, it appears that this can be true. Be patient and give it another three minutes—soon they'll be pummeling each other like every other set of siblings.

And the biggest myth of all is . . . *Twins are double trouble.*

That is absolutely *not* true. Ask any parent of infant or toddler twins . . . twins are *ten* times the trouble, but worth every effort!

Points to Ponder

What myths have you heard about twins? Can you name any that weren't mentioned above?

Do twins run in your family? If so, do you believe this "myth" to be true?

Why do you think that giving birth to twins was considered a good omen or a bad omen to certain ancient people?

Do Twins Have ESP?

For centuries, people have theorized that twins—especially identical twins—can read each other's thoughts. Unfortunately, the jury is still out on this question. Studies have failed to conclusively prove a psychic connection between twins. Twins spend so much time together, and that probably explains why they tend to understand each other's needs and wants better than others do. This is similar to the phenomenon that occurs between two people who have been married for many years. Still, anecdotal evidence abounds of the astonishing "mind reading" that some twins seem to do. Certainly, Pat Enriquez of New Jersey is convinced of a special connection between her identical twin daughters. When her girls were just six weeks old, Janine began screaming hysterically as if something were terribly wrong. When Pat and her husband couldn't detect a problem, they turned to the other twin, Nicole, and noticed that she was covered in vomit, had turned blue, and quit breathing! They quickly turned her over and cleared her airway with their fingers. Fortunately, she began to breathe again and the color returned to her face. Nicole most certainly would have died if her twin sister Janine hadn't alerted her parents to her condition. How could a six-week-old child have known that her sister was in danger? We'll probably never know, but Pat attributes it to twin ESP. Even more surprisingly, this type of ESP situation has happened more than once to her girls.

Twins Tale
BEE-ING TWINS
Pat Enriquez

When my identical twin daughters, Nicole and Janine, were approximately three years old, Nicole woke us up in the middle of the night crying hysterically. It was the kind of crying that made both my husband and me run to see what happened.

She was sitting up in her bed, crying and rocking back and forth, holding her thumb, and yelling, "My sister's finger is on fire! My sister's finger is on fire!" We tried to calm her down when, all of a sudden, Janine woke up and also began crying hysterically and holding her thumb!

When we went to Janine, we found her frantically looking for something in her bed and crying harder now than ever. All of a sudden, we found a half-dead bee on her mattress, and we noticed that Janine's thumb was becoming very hot and beginning to swell. Janine had been stung by the bee, and Nicole had felt her pain even before Janine had noticed it herself!

When things like this happen to my daughters, I realize what an incredible bond they share as identical twins. They are now in their twenties and closer than ever.

Points to Ponder

Do you believe that twins share a psychic connection? Have you seen any evidence of this with your children?

Do you think that identical twins are more likely than fraternal twins to have ESP? Why or why not?

Should Twins Share Everything—Even *Spit?*

When my twins were babies, I was determined they wouldn't share germs. I color-coded their pacifiers (blue for Caleb; green or red for Austen), their serving spoons, their bottles, and anything else that touched their lips. Much to my dismay, the minute I turned my head, they would be swapping binkies (pacifiers)! Austen would be happily sucking away on the blue binky, while Caleb had the green. It wasn't a matter of preference. If I started Caleb out with the green one, I'd soon find him sucking on the blue! If one of them had the sniffles, I'd be particularly alarmed that he'd pass his cold on to his brother. After all, dealing with one sick child is bad enough; handling two is a nightmare! When it came time to give them baby food, I would painstakingly give a spoonful to one child with one spoon, then lay it down and use another spoon for the other baby. Back and forth, back and forth we went. It was extremely tedious and took a long time to get through the meal.

Eventually, I reached the end of my patience. I realized that neither of them had suffered from swapping pacifiers, and I finally decided that one spoon would be much more efficient than two. If one baby finished his bottle and the other was still hungry, I had no qualms about giving the ravenous kid his brother's bottle. And guess what? They survived! I think this germ swapping actually built up their immune systems because they've been astonishingly healthy. Now when one is sucking on a toy and the other grabs it out of his hand and transfers it to his mouth, I don't bat an eyelash. In fact, I don't even cringe now when it's picked up from the floor and put in the mouth! (Okay, at first, I ran to wash it off, but that soon got old, too. And I still would never allow my twins to suck on something that fell on the ground outside or the disgusting store floor. I do draw the line somewhere!) But let's face it, kids unwittingly share germs all the time. Have you ever thought about how many runny-nosed kids must have played in those ball pits at the fast-food store or put their germy hands all over the grocery cart handle? You're never going to avoid germs completely.

Sure, if one twin has a particularly nasty flu bug, you should do everything in your power to try not to expose the other one. Do take the time in this instance to make sure they use separate spoons and pacifiers. Wash your hands frequently, especially after handling a sick child or changing his diaper, so you don't transfer his germs to the other child. And keep floors as clean as possible (especially if you have pets). Some diseases can be transmitted to people from animals, so don't let your twins kiss the dog.

But the moral of the story is don't be obsessive about germs with multiples. Most new parents get past this paranoia after the first few months. And, for those illnesses that are transmitted through the air, separate spoons just aren't going to be enough to prevent their spread anyway. So, if the kids are healthy and you're in your own home, I say, "Let 'em swap!" Besides, who can resist the sight of your twins planting a sweet little kiss on each other? People have been "swapping spit" for ages, and mutual affection should always be encouraged!

Points to Ponder

Would you describe yourself as "germaphobic" or are you more relaxed about germs? Has this changed since you've had kids?

Were you concerned at first about your twins "swapping spit" and sharing germs? Have your views changed as the kids have gotten older?

What is the grossest thing you've ever seen in terms of germs, such as watching a child pick up a used piece of gum from the sidewalk and eat it?

Twins Tips
HOW TO MAKE HOMEMADE BABY FOOD
Michelle Brouillette

When my twin girls were beginning to eat "real food," I would purchase no-salt-added canned vegetables and no-sugar-added canned fruits. I would then puree them in a blender, place them in ice cube trays, and freeze them. One can of fruits or veggies would usually make a whole ice cube tray. When they were frozen, I would then place the cubes in a Ziploc bag until I needed them. At mealtime, I would just pop the desired number of cubes in the microwave for a few seconds because they thaw very quickly! I only used two cubes of veggies and two cubes of fruit per child with each meal when they first began to eat real food, so a can of vegetables would last about a week frozen. This saved me a lot of money because I was able to avoid buying jars of baby food. The only time I purchased baby food in a jar was if I caught some on sale.

I learned this tip from a cousin of mine who did not have twins, but I knew right away that this is a great idea for parents of multiples because it is easy and so economical. When I began to make my own baby food, I bought some baby food from the store and compared the taste to my own baby food. It was exactly the same! I also bought the large jars of unsweetened applesauce and used that instead of buying the small individual jars of baby applesauce. This, too, was very cost effective.

Twins Tale

DOUBLE ABC
Holly Engel-Smothers

Double **A**ngels

Double **B**abble

Double **C**ar seats

Double **D**estruction

Double **E**mbrace

Double **F**riendship

Double **G**rouches

Double **H**air

Double **I**dentities

Double **J**oy

Double **K**isses

Double **L**ove

Double **M**idnight milk

Double **N**aughty

Double **O**bedience

Double **P**erformance

Double **Q**uiet

Double **R**ub-a-dub

Double **S**wimsuits

Double **T**utus

Double **U**nderwear

Double **V**alentine

Double **W**restlers

Double **X**-citement

Double **Y**ell

Double **Z**any

A Special Note for the Fathers of Twins

Dads, if you want your wife to adore you forever . . . if you want to win *huge* brownie points with her . . . if you want her to worship the ground you walk on, then you've got to read this story and do what it says! Trust me on this. You'll win the Husband of the Year Award hands down. (And moms, if you're reading this, you may want to make a copy and stick it in your husband's briefcase or inside his morning paper.)

Twins Tale

A LOVE STORY
Erika Tremper

My twin girls were so new. There I was, a not-so-young mother getting through the days and nights mostly alone. I was so busy that I often didn't remember to eat until late in the day, not noticing I hadn't eaten or so overwhelmed that I ignored the hunger signals that I am sure were there. The overriding theme of my life in those days was sleep, or more accurately, lack of sleep. Two colicky two-, four-, six-week-old infants. Two colicky two-, four-, six-month-old babies. Me, home all day while my husband worked sixty-four miles away. My own mother lived sixty-seven miles away. All of my friends lived far away and had lives and children of their own. Because of my need for a military-style routine, the occasional visit from a friend or relative eventually became more burdensome than helpful. But with sleep, ah, precious sleep, I could have been a smiling television mom. *There is nothing so hard about a baby,* I told myself. *True, it can be staggering to most new parents, but it is doable. You can rearrange your life around the new intruder, and eat and sleep and function as a normal human being.* But with twins, well, that got a little more complicated.

When I think back to the well-meaning advice I received, it still irks me. "Just sleep when they do." "Remember to have a date night with your husband." "Hire a mother's helper." My twins never slept at the same time; one was always awake and crying to be fed, changed, or rocked. Both my husband and I would have gladly traded a night out anywhere with anyone for just a few hours of sleep. Mother's helper? Even if we could have afforded it, I wouldn't have had time to interview and train anyone. And I felt guilty that I couldn't give the girls the attention—the quiet, sweet, diaper commercial, mom-and-me attention—that I longed to give each one. I was with them all day and all night, but I was always doing, never just being. Feeding, bathing, changing diapers and crib sheets, washing clothes, sterilizing bottles. I wanted so badly to just sit calmly and marvel at the wonder that was each of my new children.

My husband and I did develop a workable routine. He would come home from his job as a computer programmer around 7:00 P.M., and an hour later I would go to sleep and he would take over "baby detail." At

1:00 A.M., he would go to bed and my shift would start. I would stay awake until 8:00 that night. We were always tired, especially because we were in the process of moving, but somehow we managed to get through the days and nights—and even laugh and enjoy our new family.

One morning, when Chloe and Morgan were four months old, I awoke to sunlight filtering in through the partially opened blinds. I saw dust motes circling above the wood floors and my first thought was, *They slept through most of the night. My mother was right—it finally happened.* I was wrong. Instead, my husband had decided not to wake me for my 1:00 A.M. shift. He stayed awake through the entire night so I could get a full night's sleep.

This is my love story. No diamond or car or any other gift could have been more precious to me than what he gave me that morning. I hadn't felt so rested in over a year. He went to work that day, and he never mentioned it again, but I think of it often. I think of it when he does something that makes me angry, and I think of it when life just becomes too hard and I need to remember reasons to love him. That incident, five years ago, defined how I feel about my husband and how I hope to always feel about him for the rest of my life. No one but a new mother of twins who doesn't have round-the-clock help can relate to the utter frustration of continued lack of sleep. The point is, my husband was equally sleep deprived and he gave up his precious few hours for me.

So, this is my tribute to the man whose genes shared in creating my precious daughters. I am proud he is my husband, and I love him for the sacrifices he has made for me and them—for us. I hope my daughters have inherited his kindness and intelligence, and that they find the love that I have in this often unloving and cold world. I hope they each find someone just like their father.

Twins Tips

FATHER-TO-FATHER ADVICE
Jason Westcott

Looking back on the first year with our twin boys, I now realize that whatever I was going through, my wife was going through as well—and it most likely affected her even more. I wish I could go back sometimes and say, "How do you do it?" and thank her for everything she did. I try now to thank my wife every day and show her that she is important. Without her, I would never have made it through that first year. My advice to all fathers—and mothers, too—is to remember that our partners are going through the same emotions as we are—and in some cases, higher emotions. Take time to thank your spouse for what she does and let her know she is appreciated. This will make the stress of raising twins a little better because your significant other will know that you care about her and appreciate what she does on a daily basis.

Points to Ponder

What have you done for your spouse lately to express your appreciation for him or her?

What has your spouse done for you that really touched your heart—or what would you like him or her to do?

When was the last time you told your partner you loved him or her, or just extended a hug? (If it's been a while, do it now!) Have you ever thanked your spouse for making you a parent?

Twins Tips
FINDING QUALITY COUPLE TIME
Pam Pace

As the parents of triplets, my husband and I find it necessary to reconnect each week as a couple. The stress of going from couplehood and double-income comfort to parenthood and single-income "barely making it" can be very stressful. We make sure we don't lose sight of each other. If we do not have the money for dinner or a movie, we just get out together as a couple and go to the mall for a cup of coffee. When the babies were infants, it was easy to stay in and have a "date." Our home dates consisted of ordering Chinese food and renting a movie. This was easy to do when the babies were little, but once they became toddlers and could talk, we could barely hear each other. At that point, it was easier to have the babies in bed by the time a sitter came so that we only needed to hire one sitter at a fairly low rate.

We began using sitters around the age of six months. I found three teenagers, and we ended up staying with the most mature of the three. We paid the teenager $4–5 an hour to baby-sit and increased her pay each year. Eventually, she could put the kids to bed, and we could go out earlier. I also had a ten-year-old "mother's helper" (a neighbor) who would come over to play with the babies while I returned phone calls and folded laundry. We paid her $2 an hour. She would come every Tuesday and Thursday from 4:00–6:00 P.M., which were our toughest hours. Her parents loved that the babies kept her busy and taught her responsibility; we loved having the extra help at such a low rate. To find good sitters, ask around. Your friends and neighbors may be able to refer you.

Once a week, my in-laws would drive down to baby-sit and help me do laundry. I welcomed the help and adult interaction. They loved seeing their grandbabies and the babies loved seeing them!

For the sake of our sanity, my husband and I also felt it was important to give each other time to sleep, as well as time alone. Stephen and I took turns letting the other sleep. I was "off" every Friday night. Daddy would take the 2:00 or 4:00 A.M. feeding and I got to sleep from 8:00 P.M. until 6:00 A.M. I would have to get up and pump once, but I got so good at pumping that I could do the whole process in about fifteen minutes! Stephen would sleep in on Saturday mornings as long as he liked. We put night shades on our bedroom windows to help us sleep and nap at strange hours.

Stephen also found it necessary to relax and unwind from the stresses at home by going to the gym on his lunch hour about three times a week. He would also go on jogs often. He really needed that outlet to stay physically fit and mentally in check!

I found writing in my journal relaxing, and I loved to unwind by meeting a friend out for dinner. As tired and exhausted as I was, I needed to be able to get dressed and have some adult conversation.

It can be a difficult adjustment to go from being a couple to being a family. Just try to remember why you got married and had children in the first place! Staying in love and married is one of the best gifts you can give to your children. We found that with a little creativity, we could carve out some time together, as well as give each other some time alone. This enabled us to keep our marriage a priority, as well as be the best parents possible to our triplets.

Points to Ponder

Has becoming parents placed more stress on your marriage? In what ways?

Are you and your spouse able to get any "couple time"? If not, how can you make this happen?

Do you feel refreshed after getting some time to yourself? What can you and your spouse do to make sure you each get time alone to relax and rest?

Intriguing Twins
CELEBRITY PARENTS OF TWINS

Madeleine Albright	Mia Farrow	Julia Roberts
Muhammad Ali	Vonetta Flowers	Emily Robison
Ed Asner	Michael J. Fox	Kenny Rogers
Adrienne Barbeau	Mel Gibson	Ray Romano
Angela Bassett	Bruce Hornsby	Dougray Scott
Meredith Baxter	Ron Howard	Jane Seymour
Corbin Bernsen	Christine Lahti	Cybill Shepherd
George W. Bush	Ivan Lendl	Donald Sutherland
Justin Chambers	Joan Lunden	Niki Taylor
Beverly A. Cleary	Loretta Lynn	Margaret Thatcher
Geena Davis	Martie Maguire	Cheryl Tiegs
Patrick Dempsey	Soledad O'Brien	Esera Tuaolo
Robert DeNiro	Jane Pauley	Denzel Washington
Melissa Etheridge	Patricia Richardson	Bob Woodruff

Preserving Memories

Finding the time to document our children's life events can be daunting when we're in the midst of heating bottles, changing diapers, introducing solid foods, and trying to get some rest. With twins, it may seem nearly impossible at first thought. Sure, we can snap some pictures, but who has the time to download them from the digital camera or get them developed? We can haul out the camcorder, but the babies seem to stop their cute antics the moment the camera starts rolling. Preserving these first years definitely takes planning and sacrifice, but it's worth the effort. The following moms of multiples, Lisa Henshaw and Denice Aldrich Jobe, tell us that recording memories is possible with a little creativity and some confidence.

Twins Tips

MAKING LASTING MEMORIES
Lisa Henshaw

- I keep a journal for each of my twins and write in it as often as I can. I talk about what they did each week, funny things that happened to them, milestones, etc.

- Take pictures of family members with your children (aunts, grandparents, etc.). Make sure you make a point of getting at least one good picture of each special person in your children's lives with them at each stage of life.

- I took apart my twins' crib bumpers and made scrapbook covers out of them. They are cute and sentimental.

- When my twins were born, I had a regular 35 mm camera (not a digital camera). I made copies of each roll of film for each child and put them into picture boxes right away so they would each have a copy when they got older.

- When my twins were small, I began singing them a song about family. It goes like this: "Mommy loves Emma, Mommy loves Julian, Emma loves Mommy, Julian loves Mommy." We go through each person in the family (Daddy, Grandma, aunts, uncles, etc.). We still sing the song, only now they start telling me who loves them!

- Since some members of our extended family live far away, we have family pictures all over the refrigerator. We identify the people in the pictures for the twins and talk to them about the people (for instance, "You look a lot like Grandpa"). It also serves as a reminder of the people who have passed on ("Remember how Grandma used to sing to you?"). When the twins start talking, they'll love to look at the pictures and name everyone.

- For my twins' first birthday, I bought one small, blank book for each child and had guests write a birthday wish for each along with whatever special sentiments they wanted to add. I used craft glue to decorate the books with the theme of the party and put in pictures of the party guests (labeling each picture below it).

Twins Tale

TWINS AND A NEW HOBBY ARE BORN
Denice Aldrich Jobe

I bought my first scrapbook in twenty years out of desperation. I couldn't find the right baby keepsake book for my twin boys. I didn't know it then, but working on their scrapbook would get me through the first grueling months of parenthood. I was a new mom, exhausted and in over my head. Working on the boys' scrapbook became an escape from round-the-clock feedings, diaper changes, and Mt. Everest sized mountains of laundry. It was a chaotic, uncertain time—a time in which, like many first-time moms, I was adjusting to a new life and a new role. Motherhood brought with it a steep learning curve. Scrapbooking made me feel better. Here was a worthy, creative project I could do between feedings and during naps. Each page was an accomplishment, a piece of art I could finish in a day or two.

Before Nick and Henry were born, I searched unsuccessfully for the perfect baby book. There were only a few on the market for twins, and none of them were quite right. My ideal baby book was simple and classy, with room inside for photographs and plenty of journaling, and just enough direction, in the form of fill-in-the-blanks, for what to record in my babies' first years.

There would be a typical family tree page, pages for first-time events, holidays, and special outings, and space to write my birth story. Each child would have his own section in which I could document his birth weight and length, record his first tooth and when he first crawled, explain how he got his name, and display special mementos such as his hospital ID bracelet and cap.

For a while, I considered buying two baby books, each designed for a singleton, or two identical books packaged specially for twins. But the thought of maintaining two books and duplicating pages was overwhelming. I knew that once my twins arrived, I wouldn't have a lot of time to record their stories and milestones, and I didn't want it to feel like a chore. I wondered, though, would my sons, when they got older, complain about having to share one baby book? I puzzled over this because I wanted to treat them as individuals, not as a matched set. In the end, though, practicality won out.

I called my husband's cousin, a scrapbook consultant, and she showed me a few of the products she sold. Things had certainly changed in the years since I had last kept a scrapbook! I was a teenager then, and my scrapbook held mostly magazine clippings about Harrison Ford messily pasted on paper that definitely was not acid free. My only tools were a pair of all-purpose scissors and Elmer's glue. Now there was a dizzying array of tools: scissors that cut intricate edges, circle cutters, and photograph trimmers. I settled on a navy blue scrapbook and a set of basic tools to get started. I also bought two sets of pre-printed baby boy pages from which I planned to pick and choose to create a custom baby book.

While I waited for my order to come in, I visited the scrapbook store. I walked the aisles aimlessly, dazed. The reams of paper, the drawers of die-cut images, the tools, the thousands of stickers—it was paralyzing. I had to stop and think about what I actually needed. After that, shopping for supplies got easier. I left carrying the parts of what would become my first page.

I was so proud of that first effort. The page was blue and titled, "How many?" In the center I glued down an ultrasound picture of the twins when I was seven weeks pregnant, and under that I added an excerpt from my journal: *It's confirmed! We're having twins!* Other pages quickly followed. One page showed how enormous my belly grew over the course of my pregnancy. Another told the story of how I was confined to bed in the hospital for eleven weeks because of complications. Finally, the birth—a two-page spread I adore, and yet it fails to adequately communicate in pictures and words how astonished, relieved, and besotted we were when Nick and Henry came into the world.

I was seven pages into it, using my own ideas, when my scrapbook order came in. It was then that I realized I didn't need the pre-printed boy pages anymore. I had struck out on my own, creating my own pages, my own themes. Fill-in-the-blanks now seemed restrictive. The layouts I was most proud of were the ones I thought up on my own, like the bath-time page and the page about an infant massage class we had attended as a family.

Before beginning, I worried that I wouldn't know what to include in my boys' scrapbook. I wanted both direction and the freedom to be creative. In the end, I chose full-blown freedom. After all, I know my family best and what milestones should be documented.

Nick and Henry—and their scrapbook—have gained an amazing amount of weight in the last two years. I just finished a page about their first trip to Miami Beach. These days I'm feeling more confident as a mom. It is easier to give myself credit for doing a good job now that the fog of sleep deprivation and self-doubt has lifted. Those desperate, frenzied early months passed us by in a blur, but the images and words captured in the scrapbook will always be lucid and vibrant. I'm proud of what I accomplished. I learned how to mother twins. And I created something significant in the process, something that, I hope, will entertain and move my children for years to come—just as it moved and entertained me when I made it.

I plan to continue scrapbooking through the boys' toddler years and beyond. I like the idea of a travel scrapbook they can add to as they grow up and visit new places. I wonder, though, if I'll need to make two of them next time. As they grow older and begin to have more individual experiences, it might be the best option. With my newfound confidence as a "master scrapbooker," I know they'll both be wonderful mementos for Nick and Henry.

Points to Ponder

Have you started a scrapbook and/or photo album for your twins? Did you make one or two? Why?

Do you find it daunting to document your twins' lives due to lack of time, sleep, or skill? What can you do to overcome your hesitation?

Do you find that you're taking more or fewer pictures and videos as your children get older? Why do you think this is happening?

What other creative things have you done to commemorate your twins' milestones?

Twins Tips

HOW TO HAVE A GREAT FIRST BIRTHDAY PARTY!

I happen to be one of those moms who believe in low-key family celebrations for first birthdays. After seeing too many parents get all stressed out trying to plan the perfect party—only to find that the oblivious child hardly appreciates it—I've learned to save my party-planning skills until the kids are old enough to enjoy them. But, if you've got your heart set on a big shindig for your twins' first birthday, please keep the following tips in mind.

- Experts advise that first birthday parties shouldn't last longer than an hour and a half. Babies usually get cranky if the party drones on, and with twins the crankiness will be turned up to the *max*!

- Keep nap times in mind. Try to schedule the party for late morning or late afternoon, when your twins are well rested.

- Don't overdo the guest list. More people mean more chaos. Your children are young. They're not going to know or care if you didn't invite every kid on the street. Keep the list small and invite only those who are nearest and dearest to you and the twins.

- Have kid-friendly food on hand. Serve lots of finger foods and check with parents beforehand about any allergies. Don't serve anything that little ones can choke on, such as hot dogs. And make sure you have food for the adults, too! Make it easy on yourself and order lots of pizza or have the party catered.

- Don't stress out. With little kids, there are going to be accidents and meltdowns. The babies are going to get cake and ice cream all over their darling party outfits. Keep your cool and relax, and others will follow your lead.

- Ask someone else to take pictures so your hands are free to take care of the kids, serve drinks, etc. If you want a picture of each guest, make sure you instruct your photographer about your wishes.

- Have lots of toys and activities planned for the kids. Set up age-appropriate "stations" for play. For instance, tape big pieces of paper to the floor and supply washable crayons for little ones to color with. Set up "Pin the Tail on the Donkey" or a piñata for kids who are a little older.

- If you're planning on handing out goody bags, make more than you think you need just in case an unexpected sibling or friend tags along. Make sure the toys inside are appropriate for little ones—nothing with tiny parts that can detach and be swallowed.

- Baby proof your party place, especially if you're away from home. Put plug covers on all the outlets. Make sure that grills and hot food stations are out of reach of little ones. I remember attending a party once where the party room opened right up onto a lake. I was terrified all night that someone would lose track of their little one and find they'd tumbled into the water. Choose a safe setting.

- Take two pieces of poster board and place a photo of each baby in the middle, one baby apiece. Pass them around for guests to write a signed message to each child. These will be wonderful keepsakes of the party! Another great idea is to decorate two special containers (one for each twin) and have guests drop loving messages inside for your children to read when they get older. Guests might write "What I like about you . . ." "My hopes and dreams for you are . . ." "You're special because . . ." or anything else personal about each child. You'll love reading them, too!

Points to Ponder

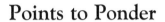

Do you plan to have a big birthday party when your twins turn one year old or celebrate quietly at home? Why did you make this choice?

What mistakes have you seen other parents make at first birthday parties?

What ideas do you have for making your multiples' first birthday special?

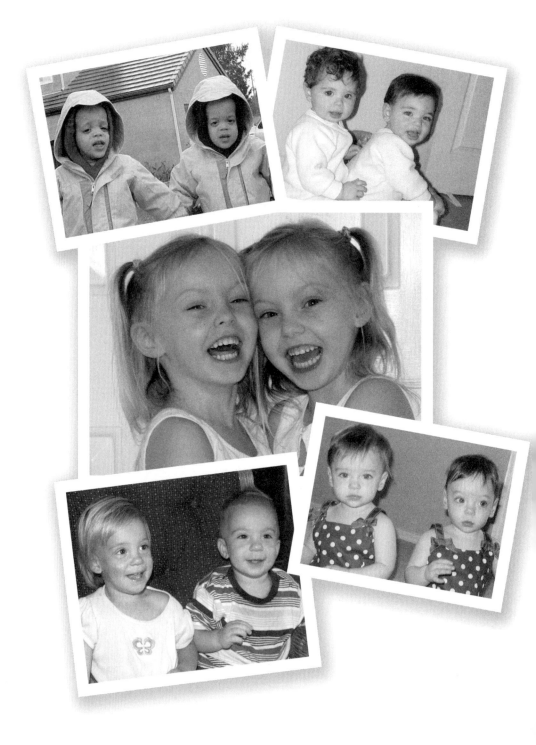

2

Twin Toddlers and Preschoolers
(Ages 2–4)

W hen I was going through the really exhausting days of infancy with my twins, I remember thinking to myself, *Boy, I can't wait until they can walk and talk. Once they're a little more independent, it will be so much easier!* Now that my twins are toddlers, I feel like a complete idiot! How could I have thought it would be easier? They went straight from walking to running—in opposite directions! They have no fear of anything. One may be climbing out of bed as the other is scaling the floor lamp. They throw everything. They have tantrums. They say "No!" to every request. They completely ignore me when I tell them not to do something. I don't mean to sound discouraging, but life is tough with these two!

Take this morning, for instance. I decided to take the boys to Kmart to shop for sandals and diapers. Caleb refused to get into his car seat until I promised to play their Winnie the Pooh movie on the portable DVD player. Once we arrived at the store's parking lot, it took me fifteen minutes to drag the stroller out of the back of the van, roll it around to each side of the car, and place each boy in it. (I also double-checked to make sure I had my purse as I was so distracted on two previous trips that I left it in the car!) Once we got inside, there was no way we could bypass the Easter display smack-dab in the front of the store, so we spent ten minutes there with the twins handling each one of the toys and me trying to pry them out of their hands without making them scream. Finally, we were ready to move on. I hurriedly made our way over to the shoe department to look for sandals for the twins. The toy department is unwisely situated on one end of the shoe department, so I attempted to stay on the opposite end to avoid having the twins glimpse the toys. Wouldn't you know? The rack of sandals I needed just happened to be on an end cap facing the toys! So, in order to get the boys to cooperate in trying on shoes, I had to promise them we'd visit the toy aisles next. Finally, we had the shoes and headed over to the toy section. That was another twenty minutes as I again wrestled with them over toys (while a store employee hovered over me, no doubt making sure we didn't break anything . . . Why is it that I can never find a store employee when I actually need help?). A few tears later (from me, not the twins), we were ready to head over to the diaper section to get that big box of diapers to juggle along with the double stroller. Unfortunately, I made the mistake of being lured in by the sign that read, "Short outfits $6." Every time we got close to a rack of clothes, Austen's little hand slipped out like lightning to pull items from hangers and sweep entire stacks of shirts from shelves. (Why do stores make their aisles so narrow? Even my one-seat-behind-the-other double stroller is too wide!) Then, both boys decided they'd had enough of looking at clothes. They engaged in an all-out fight! They were biting and hitting each other. What could I do? I couldn't yell in the store or put them in time-out. They're too big for me to carry one, plus manage a double stroller and a box of diapers. If I let them both out, they'd run in different directions. I had to keep placing my hand between them and fiercely whispering, "No!" in the hopes that no one would notice their naughtiness. Meanwhile, Austen acquired five angry red bite marks on his arm from his brother, and I was certain that everyone in the store would notice. In desperation, I abandoned my quest for clothes (which they really didn't need anyway) and headed for the checkout aisles. Naturally, only two lines were open and I picked the slower one. When we reached the cashier, Austen instantly spied the candy conveniently displayed by the register and swiped several candy bars to the ground. The aisle was too narrow for me to move the boys away from the candy, so I had to wedge myself between the stroller and the candy while they hit me in the gut as they tried to reach the candy. At last, we made it out to the car (where Caleb again fought being returned to his car seat) and headed for home (with the DVD playing, of course).

So, what was I saying about life being easier after the twins leave babyhood? Okay, toddlerhood isn't all bad. I certainly love their sweet little kisses and cuddles, the way they like to wrap a blanket around themselves like a cape and play "Super Caleb" and "Super Austen," their sweet little voices as they say "Mama" and "Dada," and the excited look they get on their faces when I agree to let them watch *Caillou*. In fact, I would venture to say that toddler twins love to alternate between being totally adorable and totally terrible. So, now that we've established the fact that toddler twins are challenging, let's take a look at some of the solutions that other parents have thoughtfully provided.

Twins Tale

IT WILL GET EASIER . . .
Marla Feldman

Recently, I ran into the mother of one of my former Sunday school pupils, who is also the mother of twin boys. We chatted a bit, and she inquired about my three-year-old twins, Sam and Emma. I told her how they were enjoying preschool and how I enjoyed my few hours of free time.

Then she asked me, "Do you find it getting easier for you?"

I looked at her in amazement and replied, quite honestly, "No, it isn't any easier."

From the time my twins were born, other mothers of twins told me that it would get easier over time. As they grew older and more independent, life would not be easy, but at least *easier*. My twins are three-and-a-half years old. I am still waiting for "easier" to come.

In my sleep-deprived state, I used to hallucinate about a time when my infant children would blissfully sleep through the night. To date, I have yet to reach that nirvana. Sam will sleep through the night for a few weeks, followed by a few weeks of awakening intermittently. Permitting him to cry it out is not an option, as he will then awaken his twin and his eleven-year-old sister.

I lived for the day when each child could hold his own bottle. Of course, when that freedom came, a new game called "throw the bottle" became the norm. "Whomp your twin over the head with the bottle" was another favorite.

Schlepping the enormous double stroller with the matching car seats was always an ambitious undertaking, especially when I was alone. Most of the time, I would just carry both of my twins in the carriers.

When Sam and Emma got too big for the infant carriers and were walking well on their own, I thought it would be easier to get them both in and out of the car, as they could hold my hand and walk with me.

Wrong.

Sam would dart away and dash around and around the outside of the van. When I finally caught him, we would engage in a wrestling match, for if I did not put him in correctly, he would jump into the front or back seat of the van. While I always won, it wasn't without sweat and tears—many times my own. He even became adept at unbuckling himself, in spite of the childproof lock over the release button!

As my darlings grew older, I thought that I would be able to slowly have a few minutes to get something done here and there, as they could entertain each other. Not out of sight, mind you, just with me in the next room, a glance away. Changing a diaper or preparing a meal in the nearby kitchen was an invitation for trouble. One day, while preparing lunch, I heard banging and ran to find my busy beavers taking their Wiggles light sticks and hammering away on the powder room door. Lots of marks now decorate the six panels. Our computer is in the kitchen, and every time I would turn my back, one of my kids was pulling the mouse or banging on the keyboard mercilessly. We had to hide everything behind the monitor until they both outgrew this phase.

I thought that life would also be easier when my twins were out of diapers and wearing underwear. It took time, but both are now diaper free except at night. But is it easier? On my wallet, yes. Otherwise, no.

Emma will not go potty when asked. Each morning before preschool or before we go out to a park or to run errands, Emma will refuse to go. I am the only mother who has to arrive at preschool ten minutes before pick-up time just to take her child to the bathroom, as she will not go for her teachers.

On our non-preschool days, it is a battle of wills to get out. I do not wish to stop at every potty in town as we go about our day, and many of the parks we visit do not have restrooms. It can take up to an hour to get Emma on the potty, while Sam is jumping up and down wanting to go and willing to leave his sister behind. We have not made it to a potty every time she has declared that she has to go. Oh, and did I mention that their favorite time to go potty is during a meal? They never have to go before, only during.

Even something as simple as taking out their bicycles and going for a ride around the block can cause a major meltdown. Sam wants to ride left, Emma right. No one wants to compromise! Is it any wonder why I prefer to stay in the house?

As my children have gotten older, their antics have gotten more daring. There have been nighttime visits to the bathroom to "paint" the sink and floors with liquid soap and toothpaste. Both have figured out that chairs can be used to grasp those once out-of-reach items. Favorite games include "hide the remote" and "hide the phone." (It's ringing, but *where* is it?)

And those childproof locks? A thing of the past.

While life has certainly not gotten any easier, it certainly has gotten more adventurous. I anxiously await what the next phase will bring. Easier, perhaps? One can only hope!

Points to Ponder

When you were struggling through the newborn days, did you comfort yourself by thinking that life would get easier as your twins got older? In hindsight, what do you think of that belief now?

What new behaviors have your twins acquired now that they're toddlers or preschoolers that drive you insane?

Do you find that your twins work together to get into mischief? What have they done as a team that has gotten them into trouble?

Do you find that the simplest things, like putting on shoes or getting in the car seat, are a major ordeal or fight with your twins? How do you handle these battles of will?

Potty Training Times Two

I hesitate to give potty training advice because, honestly, there is *no magic formula*! That's right. I hate to disappoint you, but there's no one-size-fits-all solution to potty training. The method that worked for your niece's child may have no impact on your little ones. The "new system" that everyone's trying may work wonders for others—but leave your twins cold. Some kids like their own potties; others like to sit on the big toilet with a kid-sized seat. A reward system works for some, but not for others. Some kids are trained at eighteen months; others are more than three years old. Books, videos, games . . . you name it, they're all available. They might work; they might not. The bottom line is, only you know your children and what motivates them. If one method doesn't work, move on to the next. If your kids seem particularly resistant, they just may not be ready. It may be time to take a breather.

Sometimes one twin is ready before the other. That's perfectly okay. Focus on the child who's ready and don't worry about the other one for now. Chances are, once you get one trained, the other one won't want to be left behind and will potty train quickly thereafter. Persistence and patience are really important. Take them to the potty as often as possible, but don't get upset when they don't cooperate.

My son Caleb pees on the potty almost every time I put him on it, but he still goes in his pants. Austen just sits on the potty and doesn't do anything at all. I bought them special "choo-choo pants" (with Thomas the Tank Engine on them) and they seem excited to wear them and be "big boys," yet it doesn't change their pottying behavior. Just remember, very few kids enter school not being trained. Your twins will get the hang of it—in their own sweet time!

In the meantime, it helps to vent your frustrations with other potty training parents. Twins mom Laurel Hemmig Porterfield found an online group where users discuss the trials and tribulations of potty training.

Twins Tale
HELP WANTED: WE'RE POTTY TRAINING!
Laurel Hemmig Porterfield

All my life I've prided myself on being an independent woman who generally figures things out for herself. Then I had twins.

At the time of their birth, I also had an eighteen-month-old toddler running around. I was clueless about how to meet everyone's needs and still maintain my sanity. When I put my boys to bed, I was exhausted. But I soon learned that during the time most of my friends were watching reality shows, I could tap in to the twin message boards for guidance, direction, and support.

My mother raised two sets of twins, and I often turned to her as well, but not as often as I would have liked. Our long-distance calls were expensive, and for some reason I wanted her to think I could handle motherhood with aplomb. Soon I'd made many online friends, and my days were smoother as I posted my concerns and tried the solutions posted. Now that my twins are three, I still log on to the boards and post my concerns. And I can actually respond to the moms of newborns and sound very knowledgeable!

As soon as my boys' heads hit the pillow, I'm online tapping in to my inner Ann Landers. To the twin mom who wasn't ready to transition her children to toddler beds, I passed along my trick of placing a safety pin behind the zipper on their crib tents to discourage the kids from climbing out. To another mom, I shared how we had extended the life of our stroller by having the local shoe repair shop sew in extra straps.

When the discussion about diaper rash begins, I'm ready.

One mom posted: "Ladies, my boys have a diaper rash that has lasted for over a week. I took them to the doctor, and he wrote a script for hydrocortisone cream. What do you recommend to put on their butts as one has red bumps and the other one has a red bottom? I am letting them air dry and I've tried A&D and Desitin, but it is not working. Someone said to use Triple Butt Paste, but I can't find it at Target and Toys "R" Us. Any suggestions?"

I blunder a response: "If you can keep them in an uncarpeted area, the air exposure really helps. I remember when mine got a really good case of diaper rash . . . the doctor said, 'If you would change him once in awhile, this wouldn't happen.' I felt awful! Thing is, I did change him often, and it was when he was starting solid foods, so I think his skin was just extra sensitive. I also tried all the usual remedies and we used the hydrocortisone cream, but were told to only use it for three days and not for any extended period of time. So we ended up with a concoction of Lotrimin, Neosporin, and Bactroban cream. Since then, I've used petroleum jelly as a diaper rash preventative."

Then I wonder if I've said too much—or not enough.

I see that Top Mamma has posted. She always has sage advice. Expectantly, I read her comments. "Use a good diaper cream followed by a dusting of the powder called Caldesene." And, Balmex recommends someone named Been There for advice.

From diaper rash we transition to the topic of constipation, which leads us—naturally—to the topic of potty training. This lights up the message board for the rest of the week.

"Been There," I venture, "my boys have had severe constipation in the past, so I started mixing prune juice in with their milk. Now that's the only way they will drink it! Should I be concerned?"

"Not at all," comes the reply. "It's great if you can get your toddlers to drink milk at all. Stick with something that works for you."

"Top Mamma," I type, "have you gotten your dynamic duo off Babylax? And did you ever try the Karo syrup and water as a stool softener?"

"Yes," she says. "And we've moved on to those little fiber cookies. I sure hope this stage doesn't last long. It's so painful to watch!"

Then, we switch over to the topic of potty training products. *The Bear in the Big Blue House* potty video gets four stars, as does *Once upon a Potty*. Triplet Mom asks if I have a Potty Scottie doll she can borrow, but I have never heard of it. "My boys have been too busy decorating our potty chairs with stickers and fighting over who gets to do the flushing!" I post.

Top Mamma says her kids put raisins in the pot to make her think they've gone pooh-pooh. "My kids will do anything for marshmallows," she says. Triplet Mom asks if anyone has tried the Potty Training in a Day technique.

"I don't recommend it," I supply. "It didn't work for us. I spent $40 on materials and the boys weren't ready. If they are not ready, everything is so much harder."

A newcomer to the group asks what type of potty she should buy.

"Well," I provide, "any type will do. Just make sure you have two. I learned this the hard way when one of my boys pooped in a plastic fire hat when he found out our only potty was occupied!"

"My word!" said Been There. "We never had anything like that happen at our house. I just cancelled the diaper service, put the kids in underwear, and got the job done."

That response struck me as something my mother would say, and I resolved to ask her about it, but I didn't have to. During our next visit, she asked, "How's the potty training going?"

"Fine," I said.

"Plastic fire hats and prune juice in milk . . . it doesn't sound fine!" she said.

"How did you know about that?" I questioned.

"Just a hunch," she said, smiling broadly. Then I understood that my mother had indeed "been there"!

Twins Tips
TAKING THE AGONY OUT OF POTTY TRAINING

- I prefer to have my twins train on the big potty with an adaptor seat so that I don't have to wash out a training potty, but if you decide to purchase child-sized potties, most parents of twins suggest that you get two. Oftentimes, twins like to go at the same time. You can also have a potty in two different bathrooms. Some parents move one or both potties into the twins' bedroom(s) at night so they're close at hand in case your twins need to make a "midnight run."

- To give little boys more accuracy when they stand up to pee, many parents suggest that you throw Cheerios in the toilet and make a game out of aiming for them. Some stores and catalogs even carry special floating bulls'-eyes that you can drop in the toilet water.

- Don't compare your twins' potty training progress. One might train easily; the other might not. If you compare the more difficult one with the other, he may become even more stubborn just to prove that he is different! Let each train at his or her own pace.

- In the case of potty training, bribery is not a bad thing. It's called a "motivational tool." Try stickers, treats, special pants, colorful toilet paper—anything that might motivate your twins to train. My sister will kill me for printing this, but my parents said she learned to use the potty as soon as my mother bought purple toilet paper! She wanted to use that toilet paper so badly that she trained herself.

- Don't ask your twins if they have to go. Just tell them, "It's time to go now." Chances are, if you ask, they'll say "no," and then proceed to mess their diapers. Just keep up a regular schedule of taking them to the bathroom.

- If your twins attend a day care or have a regular babysitter, make sure you coordinate your potty training techniques. It's important that your children have that consistency, no matter where they use the bathroom.

- Even if your children are potty trained during the day, you may still need to use diapers at night. Some children's systems just aren't mature enough to alert them when they're asleep. Once they start waking up with dry diapers, you can eliminate them.

- If there are a lot of other changes going on in your twins' lives—a move to a new house, a new baby, a new preschool—it might not be the best time to introduce another new thing like potty training. Save it for when they won't be distracted by other stressors in their lives.

- Never leave your children in soiled clothing to punish them for having an accident. This can cause them to develop a sore bottom or a rash, which will make them even more resistant to using the toilet.

Points to Ponder

Have you started potty training with your twins? How is it going?

If you have older kids, what methods were successful in potty training them?

Are your twins alike or different in temperament? Do you think this will affect how quickly they're potty trained?

If you've been successful in potty training your twins, describe what worked for you!

Learning to Talk:
Is It Different with Twins?

Studies have shown that toddler and preschool-aged twins are generally about six months behind other children in developing language skills. There are many theories as to why this occurs. It could be due to a higher rate of premature birth among twins, which may delay many milestones, such as the development of speech. It could be because twins learn to communicate so well with each other using sounds and gestures that they don't have as much need to learn to communicate with others. It might also be because twins' parents have less time to spend with them individually in developing speaking skills. It's also common for one twin to be more advanced in his speaking skills than the other. After all, they're two different children, and every child develops at his or her own pace. At the age of two-and-a-half, my son Caleb uses a lot more words than his twin brother Austen. Although Austen is rapidly picking up words as well, he seems to be content at times to let his brother do the talking. The good news is that most twins catch up with other kids in language development by the time they're ready for kindergarten. Parents can do a lot in the meantime to help twins develop better language skills.

Twins Tips

IMPROVING YOUR TWINS' LANGUAGE DEVELOPMENT

- Talk to your twins as much as possible, even if you don't think they understand what you're saying. Make conversation as you go along your day and tell them what you're doing: "I'm washing the dishes so they'll be clean," "I'm going to get your clothes out of the dryer," or, "I want to call Grandma to tell her about your trip to the park." You'll notice, too, that your twins will probably understand you more quickly than they are able to express their own thoughts.

- Speak clearly and slowly to your twins so they can more easily mimic you, but use sophisticated speech, never baby talk. Don't say, "Go potty?" Say, "Do you have to go to the bathroom?"

- Ask your twins a lot of questions, even if they don't answer at first. Instead of driving quietly to the store, point out the sights along the way and ask your twins about them. "What color is that car?" "Do you see the spotted dog over there?" "Are you excited about going to the beach?" They will quickly understand that you're asking them a question by the tone of your voice. (We usually raise our voice at the end of a question.)

- Read to your children a lot. Recite nursery rhymes. Sing silly songs together. Talk about the words in the world all around you, such as on road signs and storefronts. Expose your twins to speech and language in many forms.

- Don't encourage your twins to mispronounce words just because they're cute. I used to think it was adorable when one of my sons pointed out a "heli-*clop*-ter," but it's better to repeat the word after them with the correct pronunciation.

- Try to get your twins to use words for what they want. If they point to a ball and you run to get it, they will find that they don't need to use words to get what they desire. Ask them to tell you what they want, but don't frustrate them by insisting on total accuracy. If they say, "Want baba," you can say, "You want your baby?" and go over to get the doll. They'll be delighted that you understood them and will continue to use speech to have their needs met.

- Ask open-ended questions where the answer requires more than a yes or no response. Don't ask, "Do you want a treat?" Ask, "What kind of treat do you want?"

- Make sure you praise your twins when they make good use of their language skills, such as trying out a new word or answering a question. And exercise patience. It can be frustrating when they try to tell you something and you don't understand, but with a little trial and error, their communication will improve.

Points to Ponder

Are your twins developing language skills at the same rate or different rates from each other?

Do you feel your twins' language skills are developing right on schedule, or are they ahead of or behind their peers?

In what ways do you help your twins develop better language skills?

Should You Teach Sign Language to Your Twins?

When my twins began to show frustration at telling me what they wanted (because their speech hadn't yet caught up with their demands!), I began to teach them how to use sign language. Since I had never used sign language before, we bought several videotapes designed to teach sign language to young children (and their parents!). At first, the twins didn't seem to get the connection between signing and communication merely by watching the videos, but as I continued to reinforce the lessons with them through our interactions, I was amazed at how quickly they caught on. When the twins first began signing, their signs were very primitive because they didn't have the hand coordination to do them properly. But as they matured, their signs got more and more recognizable. Some of their favorite signs included "more," "bird," "cookie," "book," and "cheese" (naturally, the things they want most!). Best of all, it was wonderful to see the look of satisfaction on their faces when they knew they were understood.

Sign language is beneficial to children because it helps to compensate for the fact that they often understand language before they're able to express it well. For instance, when my son Austen wanted something from me but was unable to vocalize it, he would point to things and hum. If he pointed to the cupboard and made noise, I would have to guess at what he wanted, which got very frustrating for both of us! But, when he made the sign for "cookie" and I said, "Oh, you want a cookie?" he jumped up and down with glee because he had been understood! In fact, toddlers naturally use a crude form of sign language merely by pointing to things they want or raising their arms when they want to be picked up. Therefore, teaching sign language is just providing them with more gestures to aid in their communication. Some parents worry that if children know signs, they won't bother to learn spoken words, but I don't believe that's the case. As my children were able to speak more words, they used them in combination with their signs—it was like they were speaking in two languages!

DVDs That Teach Baby Sign Language

Baby Hands Productions:

My Baby Can Talk: First Signs

My Baby Can Talk: Sharing Signs

Kronz Kidz Productions:

Baby See 'N Sign, Volumes 1 and 2

Two Little Hands Productions:

Signing Time! An American Sign Language (ASL) Video for Children, Volume 1

Signing Time! Volume 2: Playtime Signs

Signing Time! Volume 3: Everyday Signs

Signing Time! Volume 4: Family, Feelings, and Fun

Signing Time! Volume 5: ABC Signs

Signing Time! Volume 6: My Favorite Things

Barbara Granoff and Lee Sher:

Sign-a-Lot, the Big Surprise! A "Hands-On" Adventure!

Walt Disney Video:

Baby Einstein: Baby Wordsworth First Words—Around the House

Books That Teach Baby Sign Language

Acredolo, Linda, et al. *Baby Signs: How to Talk with Your Baby before Your Baby Can Talk.* McGraw-Hill, 2002.

Briant, Monta Z. *Baby Sign Language Basics: Early Communication for Hearing Babies and Toddlers.* Hay House, 2004.

Brown, Christopher, and John Clements. *Sign Language for Babies and Toddlers.* Thunder Bay Press, 2005.

Fixell, Andrea, and Ted Stafford. *Baby Signing: How to Talk with Your Baby in American Sign Language.* Studio, 2006.

Garcia, Joseph. *Sign with Your Baby: How to Communicate with Infants before They Can Speak.* Northlight Communications, 2002.

Ryan, Diane. *Complete Idiot's Guide to Baby Sign Language.* Alpha, 2006.

Points to Ponder

Do you think it's a good idea to teach sign language to young children? What are the benefits and drawbacks for you?

If you've used sign language videos or books, which ones do you like best?

If you are teaching your children sign language, will you continue to do so after they can speak well or will you stop when they can use words to express themselves?

Twins Trivia
DO TWINS HAVE A SPECIAL LANGUAGE?

Just like married couples, your twins spend so much time together that they may develop particular code words that they use to communicate. For instance, if one calls his blanket a "bubby," the other may soon follow suit. But this tendency, called "idioglossia" or "cryptophasia," can't be classified as a separate language. Just like singletons, when twins first begin talking, they have trouble pronouncing certain words. As they pick up each other's habits of saying things, they develop their own secret code. But as their speaking skills improve, the twin language will disappear.

Intriguing Twins
MICKEY CARROLL

Did you know that one of the most well recognized Munchkins in *The Wizard of Oz* movie is a twin? Mickey Carroll is in his eighties now, but he still reminisces about his former stardom, especially his role in that classic movie.

Mickey came from a family of six children, but he was the only "little person." Even his twin sister was a full-sized person. Mickey got into show business early, singing and dancing at vaudeville shows, accompanied by his brother and chaperone Bud. In 1935, he was the warm-up act for Senator Harry Truman before he gave his speeches. He even shared an apartment with a young actor named Ronald Reagan in the late 1930s. Mickey says that Ron made a great dinner of liver and onions!

Mickey's agent Zeppo Marx got him the part in *The Wizard of Oz* for a paltry $250 a week, but Mickey wanted to break into movies and work with Judy Garland (whom he had worked with in vaudeville), so he accepted. Mickey played several parts during the eight-week shooting, including a soldier, a fiddler, and the Munchkin who tells Dorothy to "follow the yellow brick road." Because many of the other Munchkins were children or for-eigners, not professional actors like Mickey, he also dubbed in many of their lines.

The Wizard of Oz was the only movie that Mickey ever acted in. Eventually, he retired from show business and opened a company for designing and building tombstones and mausoleums. His showbiz career was revived in the 1950s when The Wizard of Oz began to air on TV once a year. Mickey often got $2,500 for each personal appearance he made. After selling his business for $2 million, Mickey is now officially retired and loves to hang out with the St. Louis Cardinals baseball team!

Grocery Shopping with Toddler Twins

If the thought of heading to the grocery store with your twins is daunting, you're not alone. Honestly, I try to save grocery shopping for when my husband or teenage sons can accompany us. My tod-dlers' grabby hands and crankiness when they don't get a coveted treat are enough to get me banned from the store. Twins mom Deanne Whiteley once feared the same on a grocery store trip. She told me, "This morning at the supermarket, I couldn't find any dou-ble seat carts, so I put Zander in the front of the cart and Bailey in the basket section of the cart. I then realized that I didn't have any-where to put my groceries, but since I was only going to get a few items, I didn't worry too much. I raced down each aisle, throwing things into the cart, and the items began to pile around Bailey. He didn't seem to mind. As I dashed down yet another aisle, an old woman stopped me and exclaimed in a loud voice that I was leaking milk *everywhere*! I looked up the aisle we'd just come down and, sure enough, a trail of milk was following me all the way down the aisle. Not knowing what else to do, I laughed and said, 'Well, at least we'll be able to find our way back around the store if we get lost!' My attempt at humor drew no response; the old woman just stared at me. I pulled out some baby wipes and began mopping up the floor before quickly realizing that this task was beyond a small packet of wipes. While I waited for a store associate, I decided to deal with the milk still dripping from the cart. As I peered into the cart, I noticed to my horror that every item and package I had tossed into the cart was open! The back of the cart was an interesting mix of milk, Band-Aids, squashed bananas, and something that looked like it might have once been a loaf of bread. 'Bailey,' I scolded, 'what are you doing? Why have you opened all the groceries?' He looked at me, smiled angelically, and said, 'I open the presents, Mama!'"

Most likely, you have a similar story about shopping with your twins! But, despite these common fiascoes, twins mom Sherri Polhemus advises that we shouldn't avoid taking our twins to the grocery store. She says, "Don't be afraid to take your twins out in public, such as to restaurants or grocery shopping. The more they are exposed to public places, the better they'll behave as they grow older because they'll already understand what's expected of them. I feel that children can be socialized in many ways, and allowing them to spend time with Mom or Dad in public is one of them. You must always plan ahead. Yes, this means working with their schedule, not yours, for the first few years. Children need to know that you respect them by keeping schedules as regular as possible, understanding their needs and responding to them, and showing patience in new situations."

Leslie Kelley-Genson makes running errands with her twins a little easier by using the "divide and conquer" method. On Saturdays, she and her husband Matt split up their list of errands. Matt heads out the door with one twin while Leslie takes the other. Says Leslie, "The one-on-one time is really nice, and it is amazing how well behaved they are when they don't have to fight for attention."

Mother of three, Holly Caldwell, wrote the following story about the challenges of shopping with twin toddlers (and a younger sibling)! If, after reading her story, you still feel you've got the fortitude to venture out to the store with both twins—and your spouse isn't willing to food shop with you (in which case you should "accidentally" forget to buy his favorite brand of beer!)—then I suggest that you carefully read the tips that follow, which will help make your grocery shopping trip as manageable as possible.

Twins Tale

THE PERILS OF PUBLIX
Holly Caldwell

My poor grocery planning had led to a total lack of milk and juice in our house and the dreaded first trip to the grocery store with all three children: three-year-old twins and a seven-month-old baby girl. *Surely it is doable,* I told myself. Publix has helpful and friendly employees. They also have those neat little carts with a two-seater car on the front and a cart in back.

Since Publix employees are so efficient at snatching up all the carts from the parking lot and taking them back into the store, parking near a cart and loading all of the kids in it before entering the store was not an option. I would have to find a space close to the store. I found the best non-handicap-designated spot and went around to the baby first. Elizabeth had fallen asleep. Should I awaken her and carry a crying baby in one arm or leave her asleep and carry the tremendously heavy combo of baby and car seat that requires two hands? I decided to take her out, but was taken aback by a terribly familiar odor. She needed a diaper change. No problem. Hannah and Jonathan were still securely strapped in their car seats, and I had changed several diapers in the van before.

After the diaper change, I held Elizabeth as I unfastened Hannah's and Jonathan's straps. I held Elizabeth in one arm and held Hannah's hand in the other, and Jonathan tried to hold on to Elizabeth's foot. We made it out of the van and safely across the lanes in front of the store. Once inside the store, we were thankful to find the highly desired cart. Jonathan and Hannah were so happy that they began whooping and running toward it. "Don't run!" I warned them. I helped them into the cart and strapped Elizabeth into the cart seat while the duo screamed, "Buckle me in, Mommy!"

Whew! They were finally in, and Hannah and Jonathan had their own steering wheels. Thank you, Publix! But my joy was tempered quickly when we were approached by a friendly employee who called himself "Grandpa" and came armed with lots of Tootsie Roll Pops. "Can they have a sucker?" he asked me discreetly. "I don't think so," I said. Then he turned to my children, who hadn't heard what we were talking about, and said, "I'm sorry, but Grandpa can't." He turned back to me and said, "Are you sure? I always ask first." Now feeling like a mean mommy who's probably just a little too paranoid about the kids choking on hard candy, I relented. "Okay, give it to them."

They chose their pops and happily "drove," licking and pointing out everything they recognized in the store. Meanwhile, Elizabeth was perfectly happy to chew on my purse handle. *Hey, this is not too bad,* I thought. *I might get some serious shopping done today.* But we had no sooner completed two aisles when Jonathan began screaming like he was in pain. He held out two hands with brown goop. "Clean my hands!" he demanded. Big tears began to splash from his eyes as I asked him to wait a minute. I rushed to the front where "Grandpa" had assured me the cashiers were equipped with lots of wet wipes and interrupted one of the busy cashiers, "The man with the lollipops said you have wet wipes up here. May we have some?" The irritated cashier replied, "I don't have any . . . oh, yes, here they are," and handed me one little towelette. I wiped Jonathan and attempted to resume shopping. Again, his demands for sticky-free hands began. I grabbed a dry paper towel from the meat aisle. It didn't remove all of the sticky goop either. Finally, I asked for wet wipes from the butcher, who gave us some wet paper towels.

At last, the kids were clean and I was able to shop for a while. We were in the final aisle when Jonathan said the dreaded words: "I have to go to the bathroom." I parked the cart near the restroom, got the kids out, and in we went, the four of us crowded into a stall, where Jonathan was able to go on his own by standing up. But Hannah (who also had to go) needed me to help her up while I still held on to infant Elizabeth. We all washed our hands and exited the bathroom. I strapped them all back in, and we made it safely to the checkout. "Grandpa" pushed the cart to the van, unloaded the groceries, and took away our cart. As we drove away, I sighed in relief. Hannah continued to lick her lollipop, Elizabeth quietly looked around from her car seat, and Jonathan exclaimed, "I want to go somewhere else! Let's go to Wal-Mart!" *No way!*

Twins Tips

MAKING THE GROCERY STORE EXCURSION
AS PAIN FREE AS POSSIBLE

- Plan the trip for when the twins are in a good mood. If you've already run several errands that day and they're tired or hungry, give it up and go home. Don't try to shop through lunch or naptime.

- Scope the parking lot for a "kids' cart"—those cute carts shaped like a car or with special big kids' seats located in the front. (If you only need to get a few items, the double stroller with a holding bin is probably best.) Get a Costco membership if you can because their shopping carts have two seats in the front—perfect for twins! When you spot your desired cart in the parking lot, park near it so you can easily drag it over to the car without leaving the kids unattended. Some stores have the carts lined up outside in front of the store. Although I don't normally advise people to park as close to the store as possible (everyone should get some exercise!), this is an exception to the rule. Park as close as you can, which enables you to quickly grab one of those carts at the front of the store without straying too far from the kids. If it's more than a few steps away, you'll need to have the kids walk with you until you reach the cart.

- If you can follow the tip above *and* park next to an empty parking spot, even better! This gives you more room for loading and unloading, and the twins won't be running their fingers all along the dirty car (yours or the one next to it!). Parking lot "islands" are also great to park next to because nobody can park beside you.

- Try to shop during non-peak hours, like Monday mornings. Avoid the weekends, when everyone is out and about. Peak times will slow you down and increase the chance that you'll be waiting in a long line to check out—a prime opportunity for your multiples to start fussing.

- When you enter the grocery store, head to the bakery first. Many stores offer free sample cookies for kids. This will usually keep them occupied for a while. I recommend the sugar cookies over the chocolate chip cookies, as they make less mess! If your store doesn't offer free cookies, come equipped with your own stash in your purse.

- Have a pack of travel wipes in your purse. Use them to wipe down the cart handles before you put the kids in, as well as to wipe the twins' hands and faces after their cookies.

- Don't leave the twins too close to the food shelves if you're wandering down the row to locate something. They'll certainly pull things off the shelf, either smashing them on the ground or putting them in the cart as a "surprise purchase." Their hands are quick at this age! In fact, it's a good idea never to leave your kids' sides for long. A tumble out of a cart to a hard floor could be fatal. More than 24,000 children had to go to emergency rooms in 2005 due to injuries from shopping carts. Make sure to use the child-safety straps.

- *Never*, ever cave in to the temptation to leave the kids in the car while you "just run in for a few minutes." The children could get kidnapped or die from overheating or you could be arrested! This is against the law and never in the children's best interest.

Points to Ponder

What tips have you come up with for making shopping with twins more pleasurable?

What is your most memorable shopping trip with your multiples?

Have your twins ever wiped out a food display or "shoplifted" a coveted item without your knowledge?

How to Cope When Your Toddlers Are Driving You Insane

Perhaps you've had more than a few days like mine. Caleb likes to pretend he's a monster and chase his brother around the room while screaming, "Roarrrrr!!" at the top of his lungs. Austen, of course, is also screaming because he's being chased. Every time I try to leave the room to get a drink or use the bathroom, they start wrestling. This time, Caleb bites Austen on the back, and Austen hits Caleb in the lip with a Mega Blok. In frustration, I put them in their high chairs for lunch. When I go into the kitchen to clean up, they proceed to throw every piece of food on their trays across the room (including yogurt!) and spit their drinks all over the floor. Do I get angry? *You bet!* I'm furious! At times, I'm nearly in tears at the prospect of another battle with them, and entirely frustrated at not being obeyed. On days like these, it's nearly impossible to keep my cool. Nevertheless, it's important to maintain the peace. The key is to ward off these episodes by having a few strategies.

Twins Tips
WARDING OFF A PARENTAL MELTDOWN

Isolate yourself from the situation. Put the kids in their highchairs or beds where they'll be safe and away from each other. Then, go into the next room and collect yourself. One day, I put the twins in their cribs and escaped to the next room to watch fifteen minutes of a comedy show I had taped the night before. The twins quit yelling after a few minutes and were happily making faces at each other afterward. Best of all, I got to do something for *me*, and the funny show lifted my mood.

Go outdoors. If the weather is decent, strap the kids in the stroller and take a walk. The fresh air and sights will clear your head, and the change of scenery will snap everyone out of their bad moods.

Use distractions. Have a few things on hand that you only bring out when you really need the twins' attention. A bottle of bubbles often does the trick! My kids love to chase the bubbles, and their giggles make me feel better. We also have a laser light that we shine on the floor and walls. The twins chase after it like they're trying to catch a mouse. It's hilarious to watch! Strap the kids in their highchairs and bring out erasable crayons or finger paints. This will occupy them for ages!

Call a sympathetic friend or family member. This may be your mom or your best friend, but call someone who will reassure you that your kids will grow up. One day you'll be wishing your children wanted you more . . . trust me! If your friend has little ones, ask her to take yours off your hands for an hour or so and promise to do the same for her the following week. Even an hour of time to yourself can be a sanity saver.

Remember how blessed you are. My first two pregnancies ended in miscarriages, and I was devastated. Every sighting of a pregnant woman (even a fake one on a TV sitcom) would put me in tears. I was terrified that I would never be a mother. Now, four children later, it still makes me giddy when I remember that my dream came true! If you experienced a difficult road to parenthood, reflect on the days when you feared you might never have children. You'll find a new gratitude for the little hellions now running around your house!

Stick in a favorite video. I know, I know, the experts say our kids shouldn't watch TV, but hey, most of those experts never had twins! I'm not advocating that your twins sit in front of the boob tube all day, but if you really feel like you're losing it, I still maintain that a half-hour of *Baby Einstein* is much better for your kids than a swat on the butt. And hey, they might even learn a new word or two!

Bribe them with food. My twins immediately stop what they're doing when they hear we're going to share a dish of ice cream! We savor every bite and stretch it out for a half-hour or so. Of course, we don't make this an everyday occurrence, but it's a sweet indulgence for a while and distracts the boys from their chaos. A word of caution: This may have the opposite effect if your twins are sensitive to certain food ingredients. Leslie Kelley-Genson and her husband Matt have found that artificial food colorings, such as Red #40 and Blue #1, really cause their boys to go buck wild when they ingest them. So, get your kids to look forward to the carrot or celery sticks!

Points to Ponder

What do your twins do that drives you insane?

What techniques do you employ to maintain your sanity?

Have you found any triggers, such as certain food ingredients or extreme fatigue, that seem to make your kids zanier than usual? How do you avoid these things?

Twins Tips

ENTERTAINING TODDLERS
Lisa Henshaw

- Before I had my babies, I would see other moms giving their little ones a lot of snacks and I vowed I would never do that! Now I say to my little ones, "Do you want Goldfish or Teddy Grahams?" The point here is that it's very difficult to keep two toddlers quiet and well behaved in a stroller while you are trying to pick out Father's Day cards. A small snack keeps busy little people focused and content.

- Washable crayons are a must. I place two splat mats (normally used under highchairs) down on the floor, one for each of my twins to sit on, and I place coloring books or giant pads of paper and crayons out for them. This is the designated area for coloring. Start this from the first time they get crayons and it will become what they expect. Also, count the crayons you hand out to your toddlers. Make sure you pick up the same number.

- I keep a basket of tub toys on the floor in the bathroom (with a towel underneath) and a potty chair on each side. When I need to use the bathroom, they play with their toys and usually sit on their potty chairs. It also helps at bath time. I tell them to pick out their toys and put them in the tub while I get things ready for their bath.

- My twins had an allergic reaction to bubble bath, but they still love to play with the bubbles. Now I give them finger paint specially made for the tub and let them play in the tub (with just a little bit of water to make bubbles) wearing only their diapers. When they are done, I rinse out the tub, take off their diapers, and give them baths. It's also a fun activity after eating messy snacks!

- I save eight-ounce milk containers and wash them well. Then I put different amounts of raw macaroni in the dry containers and screw the lids on well. We shake them and listen to the different sounds each makes. It's also fun to shake them to children's music and dance around the house.

- I have a basket full of hats, headbands, small purses, scarves, and toy jewelry. Some things fit; others are too big or too small. My twins love to pile on the mismatched items and run around the room.

Twins Trivia
ARE MORE TWINS BORN DURING A PARTICULAR SEASON?

Surprisingly, the answer is yes! In areas that experience long summer days, such as the northern parts of Japan and Finland, more fraternal twins are conceived in the month of July. It's theorized that the weather causes increased levels of the follicle stimulating hormone (FSH) in women, which affects the number of eggs that are released each month. So, if you want a second set of twins, schedule your next vacation in northern Japan in July!

Twins Tale

TWO LITTLE GIRLS
Donna Sullivan

They are twins these two
The light of my eyes.
They are too young to know
How they have changed my life.

I look at them each morning
All the wonder and glory,
I kiss them each night
Their futures so bright.

I'm taken aback by their love
And forgiving,
I'm forever grateful for
All I am given.

Their laughter, their tears
How I feel each emotion.
Their hugs and their fears
To find comfort in both.

I wake each day to find
Them together,
A mirror I see when
They look at each other.

Though one has a heart
Like a playful young bear,
The other her life
We will always beware.

They are different each one
In the way that they are,
But their hearts to each other
In harmony they are.

A love for a lifetime
For me and for them,
I was given two girls
But you see them as twins.

"Yikes! It's a Spider!"
Coping with Twins' Fears

It's extremely common for young children to develop fears. In fact, according to *The Harvard Medical School Mental Health Letter* (August 1998), 90 percent of children develop some sort of phobia. When they are very young, children usually fear real events, such as the sound of a garbage truck or a dog barking. As they mature, their fears may gradually take the form of imaginary things, like monsters, although fears of real things like insects, water, and dogs may remain. Fears are the brain's way of keeping us safe. With multiples, this problem can become compounded because one child usually influences the other. If one starts screaming about a shadow on the wall, soon they're both yelling! It's also not uncommon for one child to be more fearful than the other. One might be afraid to go down the slide, while the other goes down like it's no big deal!

Although fears are very common, they can usually be overcome with a little patience. For instance, you might want to go down the slide with your fearful child in your lap until he understands that he'll be safe going down by himself. When one of my sons was afraid of the dark, a night-light and his favorite stuffed animal "to protect him" were very helpful. Ask your child what would make him feel safe, but also set boundaries. A child who's allowed to sleep in your bed will soon be heading there every night. Let him know that he needs to find a solution in his own room.

Always take your children's fears seriously, even if they seem ridiculous to you. Even though you know there's no such thing as monsters, young children have a difficult time differentiating between reality and make-believe. If only one twin suffers from intense fears, don't allow the other twin to mock or tease her. This is a good opportunity to teach compassion. And never force your children to face their fears head-on, like throwing an insect in their lap or tossing them into the water. It's less traumatic for a child to help him overcome his fears gradually. Let your twins see you handle the things they fear, like taking a bath or petting an animal. You might try reading stories or watching videos that deal with facing fears. Try to understand where your twins' fears may be coming from. Sometimes they can spring up if a child is feeling stressed about other things, such as a new home or the illness of a family member. If they've seen a TV show or movie that has made them scared, talk about how movies are made with actors and costumes. (And do be sure to limit young children's exposure to violent events.)

Eventually, most kids outgrow their fears, but if their fears persist for an extended period of time or become debilitating (for instance, you can never take your child anywhere because he's too afraid to get into a car), then professional therapy is advised. Some children just have more cautious personalities, so you need to determine if this is your child's nature or if there's a more serious problem.

Following is a list of the most common childhood fears.

Darkness and/or shadows

Animals and/or insects

Imaginary things, like monsters or ghosts

Storms

Fire

Water

Strangers

Germs

Death (of selves or parents)

New situations (starting school, going to a party, seeing the doctor)

Falling

Using the toilet

Vacuum cleaners, lawnmowers, and other items that make loud noises

Enjoy the following story, in which Michele Christian's children freak out when they encounter a spider!

Twins Tale
THE BUG WARS
Michele Christian

I followed the rules. At age three, all kids should have their first checkup with the dentist and eye doctor, so I made the appointments, but I should have known there was nothing wrong with my children's vision. They are always able to see when their brother or sister has more Cheerios than them. They can see imaginary friends that we can't (in our house, we have "Richard"), and they can also spot bugs the size of specks three rooms away. Oh, do they hate bugs! I mean, really hate bugs! A couple of months ago, I was getting ready for work when one of my four-year-old twin girls, Emily, had to use the potty. I was putting on my makeup and nearly drew my eyeliner all over my face when I heard this blood-curdling scream from the bathroom. Emily came running out with her Pull-Ups in one hand and her dress pulled up over her head in the other. Nana was babysitting, and she ran to Emily, exclaiming, "What's wrong? What's wrong?" Emily screamed, "A *spida*!! Kill it, Nana!" Her heart was pounding out of her chest in fear. And, she didn't mean just kill it. She meant rip its legs off, pound it into the ground . . . anything! Just make it go away! Well, Nana went into the bathroom and couldn't find the spider anywhere. Emily was sitting on the couch, and Nana simply said the spider was gone. End of story, right? Wrong!

I went to work and got a call a couple of hours later. Emily had returned to use the potty. Again, she saw the beastly spider on the floor. She got so frightened that she peed on the floor and all over the spider, killing it, and then ran out of the bathroom, slipping and falling on the pee because she wanted out of there so badly! I guess it was quite a sight. I don't think she ever found out that she was the one who actually killed the spider.

I'd like to say that I have no idea where my kids get their fear of bugs, but I can't. They get that fear from me. For example, just a month ago I was working from home, and my mother's helper, ten-year-old Lauren, came to me and quietly explained that there was a *huge* spider crawling on the lampshade in the family room. I thought I'd better get it before Emily saw it, so I went into the family room and looked inside the shade. Now this spider was not only *huge*, but he was hairy and very jumpy! I so did not want this thing jumping on me! But I resolved to be brave. By then, the kids had noticed the spider and ran to the corner of the room while I plotted my attack. I ran upstairs and grabbed some spaghetti tongs—these should work, right? I also nabbed a bowl. My bright idea was to whack the lampshade with the tongs until the spider fell into the bowl. Well, I whacked it once, but then I screamed because he jumped—or maybe he didn't—I don't know! He was creepy, that's all I know. I continued my assault. Lauren, Emily, her brother Aaron, and twin sister Sara would then scream from the corner, watching every move I made. Darn it! The spider didn't fall. I had to hit it again— whack! *Aaahhh!* (that's me) and then *aaahh!* from the back of the room! This went on about five times. I remember at one point asking Lauren to get her dad or brother over here to get it for me! Finally, the spider fell into the bowl. We grabbed one of the kids' books and covered the top of the bowl, and then we all traipsed to the bathroom to watch the ceremonial flushing of the spider. Whew! We survived. That was close.

The following week, the kids had their eye doctor's appointment. Aaron and Sara successfully made it through their checkups. Time for Emily. Emily was a challenge. For ten minutes, every picture Dr. DeLugan showed her was a "bum bum." I was a bit embarrassed. I corrected her, and finally we were able to move on. The "bum bums" were gone. Next he had Emily put on a pair of 3-D glasses, and he would ask her which animals "popped" out at her. She named every one correctly. Oh, success! Then, and I should have caught this when he checked Sara, he flipped the book over and asked Emily if she could see the big fly popping out at her. Emily jumped in fright, kicked the book out of Dr. DeLugan's hand, and began to cry while ripping the 3-D glasses off her face! I turned to the doctor, smiled, and said, "Yup, she saw it. Her vision is fine!"

....

What are your twins afraid of?

How do you handle it when a child is scared of something, even if it's irrational?

Did you have any fears as a child? What were they? Have they persisted into adulthood?

Do You Have a Dominant Twin?

Has anyone ever pointed to your twins and asked, "Which is the dominant one?" or "Which one is the boss?" Surprisingly, there is very little research about the existence of a dominant twin. Perhaps it's because this situation really isn't that unique to the twin relationship—it's just more visible! Since twins are often alike in many ways, most notably in appearance, it's much more apparent when one's personality seems to dominate over the other. But when you think about it, this is often very common among siblings in general. It's not unusual to have one child who is very assertive and outgoing, while another is more passive and willing to let her sibling call the shots. Some people attribute this to birth order (although they can't seem to agree on which order produces a dominant child), but I don't believe this is a consideration when twins are born just a few minutes apart! It's just a random occurrence of personality differences. If you find that one of your twins is more dominant than the other, it's important to be respectful of their differences, yet not allow the more dominant twin to make all the decisions for both children. Never try to force the non-dominant twin to "be more like your sister/brother." This will damage his self-esteem, as you're implying that a dominant personality is more desirable. On the other hand, it's important not to allow the dominant twin to always take the reins and keep her sibling in the shadows. If, for example, you ask your twins if they'd like some ice cream and the dominant twin says, "Yes, we'll have chocolate," make it a point to address the non-dominant twin directly to ask her opinion. Make it clear that they each have a choice.

From my own experience, I've found that my twins dominate in different ways. One child is clearly dominant in speech and always jumps in with answers when I ask them questions. As a result, the other has been slower to talk as he doesn't see the need to do so! Therefore, I've been making a special attempt to spend one-on-one time with the non-dominant talker and ask questions directed only at him. We'll sit down with a book together and talk about the pictures, rather than including his twin who usually says, "Cat!" when pointing to a picture before his brother can get a word out. But my slow talker seems to dominate in other areas, especially sports. He's much more coordinated when it comes to throwing a ball or running around, while his brother has yet to develop strong athletic skills and still runs like a newborn colt just discovering his legs. Although it's easier for outsiders to notice one child's dominance in language, I'm often quick to point out my other child's dominance in other areas lest he believe his strengths are less important.

It's natural for siblings to try to assert dominance over each other, and this should be handled with twins in the same way that it would be handled with any other siblings. To recap: Respect each child's individual differences. Emphasize each child's strengths. And don't allow one twin to dominate the relationship to the detriment of the non-dominant twin. Encourage the non-dominant twin to express his own opinion without making him feel that there's something "wrong" with him if he has a quieter personality. The wonderful thing about twins is that they're never completely alike. Wouldn't it be pretty dull if their personalities were exactly the same? Rejoice in your multiples' differences and let each of them shine in their own special ways.

Points to Ponder

Does one of your multiples tend to be dominant over the other? In what ways? Is one dominant in all ways, or do they seem to shift roles depending on the skill or the situation involved?

What have you done to encourage the non-dominant twin not to be over-powered?

Should you always intervene when one twin is being dominant? Why or why not?

Twins Trivia

CAN IDENTICAL TWINS HAVE DIFFERENT HAND PREFERENCES?

If your twins are identical but one is left-handed and one is right-handed, they join the 20 percent of identical twins with different hand preferences. An ancient Iroquois legend says that the world was created by a set of twins. The right-handed twin created all the plants and animals. The left-handed twin created snakes, storms, and thorns!

Scientists aren't really sure how we develop hand preference. Most now agree that it's not a matter of genetics, as the discrepancy between twins would seem to indicate. Nevertheless, there are some interesting theories as to how we become "lefties" or "righties." For instance, some people say that the ear that faces out of the womb gets the most input from the outside world, stimulating the development of a particular side of the brain. Since twins frequently lie in opposing directions before birth, this is perhaps a plausible theory, but this thinking is flawed because it doesn't hold true for all babies.

Others theorize that increased levels of testosterone in the womb slow development of the brain's left hemisphere, which might explain why left-handedness occurs more often in males. Hormone levels also tend to be elevated during twins pregnancies, which might create more left-handedness.

Dr. Geoffrey Machin has an interesting theory in regards to identical twins having opposite hand preferences. He says that when an egg splits, the twin on the right side has to hurry to make a left side, and the twin on the left has to hurry to make a right side. This might explain why one's right brain is more dominant while the other's left brain dominates, thus encouraging them to prefer different hands.

Needless to say, researchers still don't have a definitive answer to why some identical twins have different hand preferences. It's just another feature that makes them fascinating!

Party Planning for Parents of Multiples

It's fun to create birthday parties for toddlers. They're old enough to appreciate what's going on and yet not so grown up that they've developed distinct—and differing—interests. Nicole M. Gates-Hulbert, mother of twins Brooklyn and Bheanna, suggests that parents plan a theme party for their kids.

Twins Tips
CREATING THEME PARTIES
Nicole M. Gates-Hulbert

Birthdays for multiples don't necessarily mean multiple parties, planning, and stress! Try planning a party for your multiples that will include a theme. Theme parties make it fun for all in attendance. They're great for all age groups and present a new and exciting twist that allows parents to create some meaningful memories for their children.

When planning a theme party for multiples, consider the following:

- Choose a theme that will complement both of your multiples' personalities.
- If your multiples are old enough, ask them to agree on a theme; don't impose one on them.
- Prepare to have a cake for each child, especially for milestone birthdays.
- Select a theme that can be easily carried over into the games/activities, prizes, presents, food, and drinks.

- Allow each multiple a set number of guests to keep the party controllable.

- In addition to the cake or cupcakes, create invitations and keepsakes for the guests that incorporate the theme and will knock their socks off!

- Forget about the typical commercial theme party stuff . . . *create* your own!

Are you ready to get your creative juices flowing? Plan a "Star Power" party, because at this age your children really do run the show! Have some creative pictures taken of them: Dress them up, enlarge the pictures, and put them on display at the party. Have girls wear tiaras and boys wear crowns. Roll out a red carpet and enlist family and friends to serve as the paparazzi by taking pictures of all guests as they arrive.

How about a "Picasso Party"? Lay a long roll of paper out on the driveway or sidewalk (or on the floor inside if it's winter or poor weather), as well as some washable markers, colored pencils, crayons, modeling clay, chalk, and paints. Let the little geniuses create their own masterpiece! Enhance the party by hiring a local artist to draw caricature pictures of the guests in attendance. Consider gift bags of art products for future use.

Another great idea is a "Fast Food Fantasy" party, complete with a smorgasbord of fast foods: Subway sandwiches, Taco Bell tacos, McDonald's hamburgers, etc. Set this party on another plateau by having a candy cake instead of a traditional birthday cake. (Candy cake recipes can be found by doing a search online for "candy cakes.")

As your multiples get older, they may enjoy a "Scavenger Hunt" or a "Mystery Party." This type of party allows all guests to get involved and have a great time. Prizes to the winners are the reward for being a guest at this type of party.

Planning a multiples theme party allows you to let your creativity flow. Think about your children's favorite things and create a party based around them. Everyone will remember and rave about your unique and fun birthday celebration. Happy theme party planning!

Points to Ponder

What types of things are your toddlers interested in? Do they have favorite TV shows, characters, animals, or hobbies? Are they interested in the same or different things?

What are some ideas for incorporating your twins' interests into a theme party for their birthday?

Who will be on the guest list this year?

Intriguing Twins
JOHN AND GREG RICE

On December 3, 1951, identical twin dwarfs were born five minutes apart in Palm Beach County, Florida. Their young mother named them John and Greg Rice—and then took off. Nuns and hospital nurses cared for the precious twins during their first eight months while a foster home was sought. Finally, Frank and Mildred Windsor agreed to take them in. Mildred was a devout Pentecostal and had two teenage children of her own. Mildred's Church of God family embraced the tiny twins. At one point, when they were about a year old, their birth parents decided to reclaim them, but it wasn't long before the boys were abandoned again. They were returned to Mildred's home until she died of ovarian cancer when the twins were eight. Her daughter Betty, by then an adult, finished raising them.

The Rice brothers were extremely popular at Palm Beach High School. They played cymbals in the school's band. John, the more outgoing and older of the two, had big plans for the twins. He told Greg that if they were ever going to be successful in life, "we've got to learn to run our mouths." In the 1970s, they were a big hit selling makeup door to door. When they switched over to real estate, they sold fifty-seven homes in their first year on the job. They then took on acting careers, playing landlords on the TV show *Foul Play* in 1981. Over the next twenty years, they put together forty pest control ads that they syndicated so that bug companies all over the country could adapt the commercials for their own use.

Dubbed the world's shortest living twins by *The Guinness Book of World Records*, John and Greg became international media stars, appearing on shows like *20/20* and *Regis and Kathy Lee*. The twins became millionaires and founded a multimillion-dollar motivational speaking company called *Think BIG!*

John never had his homes customized to suit his short stature. He joked that it would be discriminatory against his tall friends! He did, however, have his cars modified so he could reach the pedals. The twins were very active in their community, leading parades, speaking to schoolchildren, visiting hospitals, and hosting charity events.

In November 2005, the 2'10" John stepped off a curb and fell to the pavement. He had broken his leg and was taken to the hospital. The nasty break required surgery to repair. Sadly, John died of a heart attack as they administered anesthesia before the surgery. He was fifty-three years old. Hundreds of people attended John's funeral, mourning the loss of the little man with an enormous heart and enthusiasm for life.

When Twins Do a Strip Tease

Lots of toddlers go through a stage when they relish being naked. As soon as you turn your head, the clothes come off. Of course, this gets even messier when there are dirty diapers involved. Yuck! With twins it gets even more challenging because they can help each other strip. A back zipper can be manipulated easily by a clever twin brother or sister. There's no easy answer for this dilemma except to be patient, have a sense of humor—and, oh yeah, a roll of duct tape on hand!

Twins Tale

STRIPPER BLUES
Lori Iventosch-James

Recently, my two-and-a-half-year-old boys have taken to stripping off their clothes and diapers during their afternoon naps. It's not a big problem if you catch it pretty quickly, but it's very unpleasant if you do not! I asked other mothers of twins (MOTs) at our last meeting for advice and they recommended duct tape—yes, that silvery stuff that your husband uses in the garage. The next day, I pulled out two long strips of duct tape and wrapped them around Daniel's and Gabriel's diapers at the waist. The boys were fascinated with the whole thing and, of course, one immediately made a poop, so I had to cut him out, change the diaper, and start over. About thirty minutes later, they were having so much fun that I went into the nursery to see what they were up to. Somehow Daniel had managed to strip off all his clothes and wriggle out of his duct-taped diaper while Gabriel was wearing only a duct-tape belt with the diaper hanging from the back like a tail. Two points for Daniel and Gabriel; zero for Mom.

Next, I tried pinning their clothes on them: one pin in the front and one pin in the back. It seemed like a good idea at the time. Daniel managed to stretch his elastic-waist shorts down over his legs and tear off the diaper so that the shorts were wadded up between his legs like a thong. Another point for Daniel; zero for Mom.

I decided I just needed more ammunition. I tried two pins in front and one in back. It would have worked well except I forgot that their shirts had buttons. Daniel unbuttoned the top and then slid the whole outfit off (including his diaper). Another point for Daniel; zero for Mom.

My next idea was to put them both in zippered PJs for their naps and pin the zippers closed. (Some MOTs suggested putting on the PJs backwards so the zippers are in the back.) So far, this method has worked like a charm, but given my track record (and those of Daniel and Gabriel), I am not optimistic! I'm already waiting in the wings with Super Glue!

Points to Ponder

Are either of your twins "strippers"? What tricks have you found for keeping their clothes on?

In what ways have your twins cooperated with each other to get into mischief?

Hugs, Not Hits

I don't remember my singletons hitting as much as my twin toddlers do. Perhaps it was because my older children didn't have such a convenient target. Austen and Caleb seem to hit (or bite or scratch or pinch) each other about every fifteen minutes. It's usually the result of a toy war: whatever one child has is instantly attractive to the other child, even if a similar toy is offered. This is the typical routine: Twin A is playing nicely with a toy. Twin B runs up and grabs it. Twin A yells, "Mine!" and grabs it back. Twin B reclaims it, and then the two struggle back and forth with the toy between them. Twin B finally wins the war, so Twin A whacks him in the back as he's running away with his prize!

This scenario repeats itself over and over in my house. I used to throw a fit when I'd see them hitting each other. I'd yell, "No hit!" and take the toy away, banishing the hitter to a time out. But, sure enough, not five minutes after detention ended, another fight—and more hitting—ensued. I knew I had to come up with a new approach. Now, instead of telling them not to hit (since they don't seem to understand why it's wrong), I'm working at redirecting their behavior. Every time they hit, I take their hand and say, "Nice" and show them how to rub each other's arm or back. Whenever I see a fight in the works, instead of waiting for it to escalate to hitting, I repeat the "Nice" routine. It's gotten to the point where I can just say "Nice" at any time and I'll see one reach out to gently place his hand on his brother's arm. I use a similar technique when they try to hit me. Instead of lashing out at them when they hit me, I swallow my anger and say, "Hug." Then, I gather them close to me until they've calmed down. Amazingly, their fits of anger are getting shorter and shorter. (It also does wonders for my own temper!) The next time your twins start hitting, try redirecting their behavior. You may not notice an impact the first few times, but practice makes perfect. Be persistent in showing them how to play nice and give hugs—not hits!

Points to Ponder

Do your multiples fight with each other? Do they hit, bite, pinch, kick—or all of the above?

How do you handle the situation when they demonstrate this behavior? Does it work?

Do you remember fighting with your own siblings as a child? How did your parents handle it? Do you agree with their methods?

Twins Tips
GET A GOOD (PADDED) BRA

Dear moms of twins, you probably think this piece of advice belongs in the baby section of this book. It must have something to do with nursing, or perhaps support or sagging, right? Well, those all may be practical uses for a good bra, but the most important of all involves . . . *protection!* Think padding, moms, and the more the better! I can't begin to count the number of times those little twin elbows and knees have sent me into spasms of agony when they've stabbed my very tender premenstrual breasts. And I'm sure my toddler twins aren't the first to play the game, "Bruise the Mommy." In fact, if it wouldn't have made me a social outcast outside the soccer field, I'd invest in a good set of leg, arm, chin, and mouth guards, too. (As I write this, I am just recovering from the fat lip I received when Caleb's hard head connected with my mouth.) And these days, shorts and dresses are reserved for in-house use only, since bony toddler limbs have made a network of bruises up and down my legs. Oh, we love it when they want to crawl on our laps for a big hug, but at what age, we wonder, do they learn the art of climbing *gently?* So, mommies, invest in the best padded bra you can find! The bonus is, you'll have the best silhouette of your life!

Learn to Accept Less Than Perfection

When you have twin toddlers, you're going to have to accept that your standards may need to be lowered a bit. If, pre-twins, you made a gourmet dinner each night, you'll most likely find that it's much more practical now to heat up fish sticks and macaroni in a box. And, if you once ironed your clothes the minute they came out of the dryer, it's time to institute the iron-as-needed system. If your house was once a showcase, don't even think that you'll be able to maintain it without confining your children to one room. It's time to reorder your priorities. Accept that your kids come first and the house comes second. If you can afford a cleaning or laundry service, go for it! If your hubby's been less than helpful around the house in the past, it's time to have a *talk!* Most of all, don't let a little dirt stress you out. As I write this at 3:00 in the afternoon, I have a load of clothes in the washer, another in the dryer, no plans for dinner, and crumbs from lunch still on the floor. And you know what? I don't care! Some day I'll have an empty and very clean house, but it just won't be as much fun—or as fulfilling. Do what you can and don't stress about the rest. Mom of twins, Marla Feldman, has learned this lesson well. Read on.

Twins Tale
A BEAUTIFUL HOME
Marla Feldman

"She used to have a beautiful home."

That's what my girlfriend told another woman at our table during our weekly Girls' Night Out.

The home she was referring to was mine.

She used to have a beautiful home. The words sounded harsh coming from my friend, although it is something I had said many times over the past two years.

She used to have a beautiful home. Yes, I did. I enjoyed entertaining friends for lunches and play groups, backyard barbeques, and family gatherings.

Our firstborn, Payton, arrived nine months after we moved in. She was a good child—no drawing on the walls or jumping on the furniture. When we said "No" or "Don't touch," she listened. I had Roseville Pottery and crystal candy dishes in our family room and she never touched them. Our marble fireplace never had sets of tiny fingerprints as decoration. In fact, we always used our fireplace, even when Payton was a busy toddler. My home continued to look like new.

Unlike my friends, who were fortunate to have their second children exactly when they wanted to, I was not. As Payton grew older, my husband William and I were able to buy new couches, replacing the ones we bought when we first were married. The "Barbie Room" became what it was supposed to be: a dining room. A sunroom was added. We finished the basement and stored all things "baby" away.

Yes, I had a beautiful home.

Everything people saw, inside and out, was beautiful. But among the beauty, there was sadness. William and I had always wanted at least three children. After many years of trying, I had come to the conclusion that I did not want a pregnancy . . . I wanted a baby. So we chose adoption to increase our family.

Fast forward two-and-a-half years. Our home remained beautiful. Payton's toys were relegated to her basement playroom and her bedroom. My kitchen counters remained uncluttered. Our house belonged to us, but not really.

Every day, I anxiously awaited news from our adoption agency that a birthmother had selected us to parent her child. No such news arrived until a brilliant October day. A set of premature boy/girl twins, born at twenty-eight weeks and each weighing a little more than two pounds, was available if we wanted them. Did we ever! So, in an hour's time, our family of three increased to five—and so much had to be done to get ready for Sam and Emma's homecoming! A second of *everything* was needed. But we were never really able to get fully ready. Sam and Emma, our miracles in every sense of the word, were discharged from the hospital five weeks earlier than expected.

Entering our home on that cold November evening with two car seats, two apnea monitors, two nervous parents, and one overwhelmed big sister, our home immediately began to change. There was simply not enough room for two of everything and our family room furniture.

Out went the coffee table and in came snack tables to set the two apnea monitors upon, located directly next to the two bassinets. A nearby diapering area was established for the twenty-plus daily changes. Our fireplace was now adorned with a huge, white wicker basket full of spit cloths, bibs, receiving blankets, and assorted clothing. The two play mats joined the bouncy seat. There was little room to move. Ever present was a white laundry basket of the twins' clothing, and mine. We all changed at least three times a day.

I knew my house really looked different when a friend of mine came to visit and to meet our newest additions. She looked into the family room and kitchen and said, "In all the years that I have known you, never have I seen your house look like this!" It was honest and true. Chaos had taken over.

Our sunroom became a holding area for all of the big equipment we would eventually need. The once beige rug became spotted with endless drippy bottles, spit-up, and jarred food that spilled or was flung from a spoon. As Sam and Emma became mobile, fingerprints on the sliding doors, the TV, and the fireplace glass became my new artwork. The remote controls had to be put on top of the television and we had to remove all of the CDs from the holder, as Sam and Emma found it amusing to remove the cases and CDs and fling them about.

The pleated shades in all of our rooms had to be put permanently in the upright position, as Sam liked to squeeze and pull on them. He liked to play Tarzan and swing from the tassels on our living room drapes. "Unplug the Lamp" was a new game my kids invented to drive us insane. And, I am not sure who was teething at the time, but two of our long-awaited dining room chairs have teeth marks!

When I would tell people of Sam and Emma's latest tales of destruction, they invariably would ask, "Why don't you put up gates?" We did. Sam climbed over them!

After Emma and Sam's one year checkup with the neonatologist, it was discovered that Sam was having some problems. An evaluation by our state's Early Intervention program recommended occupational therapy. The therapist suggested equipment for Sam to climb to gain upper-body strength. My husband purchased a Little Tykes Step 2 climbing system and placed it in our family room.

The kitchen also fell victim to my twins' antics. My clever little boy figured out how to undo all of the safety locks, so we had to install magnetic ones after he and his twin sister emptied every cabinet and drawer within reach. All of the knobs had to be removed from the stove, as Sam could get them off—even with the safety locks in place! One of Emma and Sam's favorite games was "Hansel and Gretel." When I managed to get something in the oven to cook, one or both would go to the oven door to open it and hold on for dear life as they fell backwards to the floor, banging their heads. My husband put a black elastic cord on it to keep it closed. It was only a matter of months before Sam figured out how to undo it. We kept our garbage pail on the counter for more than a year, as there is nothing so much fun as digging through smelly garbage when Mommy and Daddy are not looking! The pantry, as well as every other door in our home, has extra locks that cannot be opened by Sam or Emma . . . yet.

To date, the other damages have included the following: breaking the speakers in the television, pulling out half of the slats in our verticals, peeling off wallpaper, drawing on walls, poking holes in our kitchen table with forks, ripping apart cushions and unstuffing them, and spilling nail polish all over my bedroom rug . . . to name a few.

My house will someday recover from Sam's and Emma's antics. I constantly keep in mind that things could have turned out differently. The sound of their infectious laughter could be replaced by silence if we did not say yes to that phone call. Sam and Emma could have had myriad health problems that are associated with such tiny preemies. My house could have medical equipment instead of beat up couches and crayon covered walls.

So each night as I tidy up before bedtime, I look at my children's portraits that adorn our walls. Payton, Sam, and Emma live in a house where they can be kids. We do not fret over the mess. All three are happy and healthy.

And I think to myself, *Yes, I have a beautiful home.*

Points to Ponder

How does your home differ now from when you didn't have multiples? What changes have taken place?

Do you feel you have "lowered your standards" a bit in terms of cleanliness and orderliness now that you have children? How do you feel about this?

What damage have your twins managed to inflict in your home? What creative ways of keeping them under control have you implemented? Have they worked?

Making Your Home Safe for Busy Toddlers

I had a mother tell me once that she never had to safety proof her house because she just had to shake her finger at her daughter and say, "No, no" and the little darling would just back off right away. I could only think that her child must be a robot! My charming boys have become immune to my yells of, "Get out of there right now before I put you in time-out!" They just give me innocent little smiles as if to say, "Sure, you will, and even if you do, I really don't care!" And with two, it seems that I'm always trying to get one or the other (or both!) out of trouble. From the stories I receive from other parents of multiples, my toddlers aren't the only troublemakers. Multiples especially seem to have a propensity for exploring every nook and cranny of the house, scaling every wall, dismantling every appliance and locating every hazardous product. And they usually show a great talent for dragging each other into mischief. So, it's especially important that you make your home as safe as possible.

Twins Tips

KEEPING YOUR TWINS SAFE FROM HARM

- Keep all medications, cosmetics, cleaning products, and sharp objects in locked drawers or cabinets.
- Put latches on toilet seats. Believe it or not, small children can drown in just a few inches of water!
- Clean well under furniture and seat cushions for small items that children can choke on.
- Secure bookcases to the wall.
- Make sure window blind cords are tucked up out of toddlers' reach.
- Use safety plugs on any open electrical outlets.
- Run electrical wires behind furniture.
- Keep refrigerator magnets high enough so toddlers can't get to them.
- Use appliance locks on your oven, dishwasher, refrigerator, dryer, etc. Don't let your children play nearby when you're loading the dishwasher.
- Use drawer locks on all drawers throughout the house, not just in the kitchen.
- Keep knife blocks away from the edges of counters.
- Always cook on the back burners so toddlers can't pull down hot pans. Turn pot handles to the side.
- Use corner bumpers on the sharp edges of furniture and fireplaces. (Ideally, purchase furniture with rounded edges.)
- Remove the rubber caps from door stoppers.
- Keep wastebaskets in a locked cabinet or have a secure lid.
- Keep potted plants out of reach. Some plants are poisonous and toddlers love to play in the dirt.
- Use gates in front of stairwells and in the doorways of any rooms you want your children to stay out of.
- Watch your children carefully at other people's houses. When people visit your home, make sure their bags and purses are out of toddlers' reach.

- Strings or ribbons longer than six inches should be put out of reach.
- Use the safety belts on highchairs, booster seats, and grocery carts.
- Keep furniture away from windows and keep windows locked.
- Make sure your smoke alarms and carbon monoxide detectors are functioning.
- Keep firearms and ammunition locked away and out of reach.
- Turn down the temperature on your water heater so twins won't get scalded.
- Install carpeting on stairs and secure rugs.
- Keep cribs and beds away from blinds and electrical outlets. Use side rails on beds.
- Make sure you have ground-fault circuit interrupters on outlets by sinks and tubs.
- Don't allow your children to play with plastic bags or to put them on their heads.
- Keep the phone number for your local poison control center on the refrigerator.
- Don't let kids play on the lawn for forty-eight hours after it's been fertilized or treated with pesticides.
- Never mow the lawn or use power equipment when children are around.
- Install a childproof, locked fence around the swimming pool.
- Keep latex balloons out of reach of children; they pose a choking hazard.
- Never leave your children alone with your pets, even if they're friendly.

Points to Ponder

What close calls have you had with your twins when they've put themselves in danger?

What safety precautions have you taken in your home? What do you still need to do?

Do you worry about your twins' safety more now that they move around so well? Are you concerned that other caretakers might not be as vigilant around your children?

Intriguing Twins
ANN LANDERS AND ABIGAIL VAN BUREN

For many years, it seemed as if every newspaper in the United States carried the advice column of either "Dear Abby" or "Ann Landers"—or both! They were the world's most famous twin advice columnists, with legions of fans from coast to coast. Sadly, this created a lot of competition between the sisters, and it put a strain on their relationship for the rest of their lives.

Pauline Esther Friedman (nicknamed "Po-Po") and her identical twin sister Esther Pauline Friedman (nicknamed "Eppie") were born seventeen minutes apart on July 4, 1918, in Sioux City, Iowa, to Russian Jewish immigrants Abraham and Rebecca Friedman. The twins attended Central High School, graduating in the class of 1936, and then attended Morningside College until their double wedding in 1939. They were both housewives until Eppie moved to Chicago. At that time, a family friend, Wilbur Munnecke, executive manager of Field Enterprises, informed Eppie that the *Sun Times* was searching for a replacement for its advice columnist, Ann Landers. Esther was intrigued, applied for the job, and got it, taking over the twelve-year-old column, as well as its name. Eppie's sister Po-Po soon convinced the *San Francisco Chronicle* to let her write her own advice column. From then on, she became known as Abigail Van Buren (or "Dear Abby"), and the famous rivalry between the twins began.

At the age of eighty-three, "Ann Landers" died of multiple myeloma. She left behind her daughter Margo (who has her own advice column), three grandchildren, and three great-grandchildren. As of this writing, Abigail Van Buren suffers from Alzheimer's disease. Her famous column now continues through the wisdom of her daughter Jeanne Phillips.

The Daily Feeding Frenzy

I've just finished giving my toddler twins their breakfast. I feel like I've run a marathon! And I have to do this "meal thing" how many more times today? I have this theory that most moms of twins are undernourished because they just don't have time to feed themselves! Take this morning, for instance.

"Are you hungry?" I ask Austen and Caleb. As soon as the word "hungry" is out of my mouth, they're jumping up and down wanting to be fed. Now, wanting to be fed is not the same thing as wanting to be in their highchairs. When I pick up one twin, the other howls with disappointment that he's being left behind. When I put one in his highchair, he wiggles around so that it's almost impossible to get the straps fastened around him. He hasn't quite made the connection that no highchair means no food. I finally get both twins safely in their highchairs, but they want no part of the bibs. They push their heads far back against the chair so I can't possibly get my fingers behind them to tie the bib strings. It's push and pull until finally both bibs are securely tied. Then, they lift up their knees as they see the highchair trays coming toward them. It's a game to them! I can hear their little minds working . . . "If we keep putting up our knees and placing our hands on the side of the highchair, Mommy won't be able to put this confining tray on us!" Struggle, struggle once again.

Finally, the twins are ready to eat breakfast. I decide to give them some cold cereal to munch on while I make their oatmeal. I pour some cereal on their trays, head to the kitchen, and take out the oatmeal box. "Waaaah!" They've both stuffed all of the cereal into their mouths all at once and now it's gone. I pour more cereal. Things are looking better. I return to the kitchen, make the oatmeal, and get back to the twins only to find Cheerios everywhere! No wonder they've been so quiet. They've decided to play "Toss the Cereal" to see who can throw it the farthest!

In the meantime, the oatmeal is still too hot to serve, so I give them each a sippy cup full of juice to occupy them. Austen takes a sip and then tosses his sippy cup. Caleb, not wanting to be left out of the fun, also tosses his cup. It lands on my little toe, and I'm in excruciating pain! I double over, which puts my eyes in the range of my feet so that I can see my little toe swelling to twice its size! Finally, the pain begins to subside ever so slightly and I hobble over, tears in my eyes, to pick up the sippy cups. Of course, the "spill proof" pieces inside have come out (why can't they make a spill-proof cup that works?), and juice has spilled all over the floor.

At last, it's cleanup time. As I approach the twins with a wet cloth, Caleb begins to shake his head from side to side. He hates to have his face cleaned! I sneak a swipe of the cloth in here and there as he brings his hands up to his face to avoid it. Finally, I feel he's clean enough (although I continue to find bits of oatmeal in his hair throughout the day!), and it's Austen's turn. He grabs the cloth and begins sucking on it. He's got a mouth full of teeth, and he's not letting go! I give up and get another cloth. Mission accomplished! I lift up Austen, also known as "The Hoarder," and find that half his breakfast has been shoved into his seat on either side of him. The pieces in his lap now tumble to the floor . . . another cleanup job for Mommy!

After an hour of chaos, the twins are fed and happy. It takes me another half-hour to clean the floor, scrub down the highchairs, and rinse the trays in the kitchen. Now it's time to change my little toddlers out of their pajamas and into their clothes . . . oh dear, I'd better prepare for another battle!

Twins Tips
SATISFYING DIFFERENT PALATES AND PICKY EATERS

My twins are as different as night and day, and this certainly extends to their eating habits. Austen will eat almost anything; Caleb will eat almost nothing! Austen prefers salads, green beans . . . healthy foods. Caleb eats anything with the word "chocolate" in it. I can't complain because Caleb is a lot like me: I'm also not a big greens eater and I love chocolate! I take pleasure in informing my vegetable-loving husband that our twins' differing preferences *prove* that tastes in food are genetic. After all, both twins are being raised in exactly the same way and offered the same foods, and yet they prefer different things. (Alas, my husband still thinks I'm just stubborn.) Anyway, how do you please twins with differing palates, especially if one or both of them are categorized as "picky"? Here are some suggestions:

Sprinkles: They go great on everything! I let my boys put sprinkles on their applesauce, yogurt, pancakes, mac and cheese, veggies . . . whatever they want! Somehow everything looks a little more appealing to them with sprinkles on top!

Dipping sauces: I put little piles of ketchup, mustard, and barbecue sauce on their plates and pronounce them "dipping sauces"! They have fun dipping their food in the various condiments and are more apt to eat them, as well. You can also cut up raw vegetables and serve them with a small bowl of ranch dressing for dipping.

Finger foods: Anything they can pick up with their fingers is considered fun. Cut sandwiches into little triangles. Let them eat green beans with their fingers.

Smoothies: Kids love to drink smoothies (call them "milkshakes" if you must) and they're a great way to get a good serving of fruit into your twins. Mix various fruits like bananas, strawberries and other berries, and peaches in the blender with some milk and ice, and they'll drink them up!

Individual portions: For some reason, children like having their own individual servings. Witness the popularity of pudding cups! (Well, maybe the chocolate has something to do with that . . .) Make mini pizzas out of bagels or bread slices. Serve carrot sticks in cupcake liners. Cook your lasagna in little, serving-sized pans.

Let them help: When they help you make their food, children develop more of an interest in it. I put crackers and squares of cheese and lunch meat on their trays and let them build their own sandwiches. Let them sprinkle cheese on their pizzas or make faces out of pepperoni.

Be patient: Just because your kids don't eat something the first time doesn't mean they won't try it on the second or third attempt. Experts say it sometimes takes up to ten attempts before a child will try a new food! Pick another day to serve them a food they didn't eat the first time. You might be surprised to find that they just weren't in a "new food mood" on the first (or second or third!) day.

Call it "cake": Labeling is very important. When we serve our twins banana bread, we called it "banana cake." Somehow the thought of dessert makes them more eager to try it! Call a hamburger patty a "hamburger cookie." Call it whatever you need to in order to make it sound appealing!

Don't force anything: Trying to force your toddler to eat something will only frustrate both of you. He'll just spit it out or throw it on the floor! Leave it in front of him for a while, and if he still refuses to taste it, take it away. But don't bring him a cookie because you're concerned that he'll starve! You don't want to teach him that he can have whatever he wants. He's not going to starve if he misses one meal, and he'll be that much more hungry at the next one!

Bribery rarely works: We've tried the old line, "Just eat two bites for Mommy and you can have a cookie!" It never works. It just upsets the toddler even more because he knows there's a cookie waiting in the wings and he doesn't have it!

Be the example: Let your toddlers see you enjoying foods. Show them how much you enjoy eating a carrot by saying "Yum, yum" as you eat it in front of them. Teach them that eating is enjoyable.

Check with the doctor: If you're still concerned about your twins' poor eating habits, consult their pediatrician. He or she may suggest that you supplement with a multivitamin. (Hint: My twins love those gummy bears vitamins!) Chances are, if your children are growing appropriately for their age, you don't have to worry about their diets. Kids are self-regulating and will eat when their bodies tell them they need to.

Is mealtime chaotic at your house? Describe a typical meal.

What are your twins' food preferences? Do they like the same or different things? Is it frustrating trying to accommodate their tastes?

What tricks have you discovered for getting your kids to eat their food?

Dressing Twin Toddlers

You have to be in excellent shape to get twin toddlers dressed. First, you have to chase one of them down. Once you catch him, you have to figure out how to hold him down long enough to get his clothes on. Finally, he's dressed! He darts off as you chase down the other one. While you're dressing the second child, the first one proceeds to pull off his socks or any other piece of apparel he can possibly shed. It's a vicious circle of dressing, undressing, and dressing again (and again and again).

Toddlerhood is also a time when children develop their own tastes and preferences. Some parents don't think it's a good idea to dress twins alike, but there's a good reason for doing so: If you select two different outfits, your toddlers will inevitably both prefer the same one! Even if the outfits are very similar, just different in color, you won't be able to fool them into thinking they're equal in desirability. Dressing both children exactly the same just helps cut down on the battle over which outfit is "better."

Long gone are the days when you could dress your cute little twins in whatever clothing you desired. Now they have opinions of their own, and they're determined to have their way! Mom of twin boys, Mary Brauer, discovered that dressing twins gets especially complicated when winter demands more layers of clothing.

Twins Tale
BATTLE OF THE BOOTS
Mary Brauer

The freshness of newly fallen snow blanketing everything in soft white captures something in everyone's soul. Smelling the crisp air, catching snowflakes in your mouth, and watching children and animals frolic conjure up images from our own childhoods.

As our twins became toddlers and could walk on their own, I was excited to share the experience of playing in the fresh snow with them. We hadn't had much snow that year, but at long last, the extended forecast called for a big winter storm that would arrive in three days.

I checked our supplies of milk, food, and assorted winter items. The snowsuits they received that year from their grandparents were hung in their places in the closet. Mittens, hats, and socks were all accounted for. I searched for their boots and realized after tearing apart every closet and strewing the contents throughout the house that we hadn't bought them boots yet . . . and it was already February.

I tried finding some boots online, but I couldn't find any that would arrive quickly enough. So, I packed up our twin boys and hit the stores. Store by store, we searched for any sign of boots next to the sandals and beachwear already displayed. After all, it was time for the spring fashions to hit the stores!

We ended up at a semi-famous retail bargain outlet and found the last two paltry looking boots on the racks. They were three sizes too big. Ever optimistic, I searched in vain for a salesperson on the floor. I finally caught a glimpse of one and began to barrel after her, pushing the double stroller in front of me. She noticed we were coming, spun around, and began to walk faster the other way. She was most likely terrified of either being run over by a double stroller or by being cornered and asked a fusillade of questions.

With sheer perseverance, I caught up to her and pinned her against the wall with the stroller filled with overtired and cranky toddlers. Shouting over the cacophony of the twins, I asked if they had more boots for sale, perhaps in the back room.

Suddenly, the whole store was still with shocked silence as everyone gawked at my ridiculous request. Boots in the winter? The salesperson looked at me incredulously and told me that most of the winter boot selection was sold out by the end of August. I didn't really expect to buy boots in the winter, did I?

Feeling foolishly naïve, I snagged those last two pairs of boots even though they were a few sizes too big. I rationalized the purchase by arguing that these boots would fit my twins when they reached kindergarten. In the meantime, I'd layer socks on my kids' feet to fill the gaps. Shoppers and employees were still shaking their heads as I hurried out of the store.

At last, the snow arrived, complete with all its anticipated magic. As it clung to the evergreen boughs and rapidly accumulated on the ground, I dressed myself in layers and shrugged on all my snow gear. I knew that once the boys were dressed, they would dart out the door, scattering in different directions, which would leave me no time to fully dress myself for the cold outside.

They willingly let me put on their new snowsuits, hats, and mittens. I pulled out their boots and sat on the kitchen floor to put them on my twins. I reached for the child on my right and struggled to get the first boot on his right foot. I didn't realize how difficult it is to put on someone else's boot for them. I finally succeeded in getting it on him. I picked up the next boot, which was also a right boot, and proceeded to twist, pull, and tug that boot on the other boy.

Wiping away the sweat that had accumulated on my brow, I picked up a left boot and turned to the first child. Amazingly, he had already kicked off the first boot! I huffed and puffed and returned the first boot to his foot, turned around, and noticed that the other twin had also extracted his only boot! I alternated tugging on boots, trying to beat them before they could shed them again. The heat of the house, coupled with the multitude of layers of clothes on my body and the physical effort of twisting and tugging boots onto reluctant recipients, drenched me in sweat. I figured in my daze that I had shed more calories than if I'd been on the Atkins diet.

After twenty minutes of contorting, both boys had boots securely on their feet. I hustled them toward the door and then caught the whiff of a familiar odor. Heart sinking, I sniffed both and found the culprit. I brought him upstairs to strip off the boots, hat, mittens, snowsuit, shirt, pants, undershirt, and diaper. After changing him and wrestling to put on all the clothes, which at this point he was arguing heavily about, we returned downstairs to try again to go out. Not surprisingly, the other twin had shed his mittens, hat, and one of the infamous boots.

Ten minutes later, we were outside in the snow. The snow falling on their eyelashes made them cry as they sat in one spot. After a few minutes of tears, we tromped back inside and shed all of our encumbrances. I'd lost track of the time; it was past their naptime. As I tucked them into their cribs and crawled into bed myself, I realized that it took a total of thirty minutes to get dressed for three minutes outside. It was going to be a long winter . . .

Points to Ponder

Do you think it's okay to dress twins identically or should they always be dressed differently? Why?

Do you have any "dressing issues" with your children, such as their desire to be constantly naked or their insistence on picking out their own, unmatched outfits?

If you buy different clothes for your kids, do they inevitably both favor the same clothes and reject the others?

Heading to Preschool

Going to preschool is a big step, both for your twins and for you! Some children look forward to preschool and make the transition easily. Others take some time to adjust. Typically, if you've been home with your twins up to this point, you may be the one suffering from separation anxiety when your twins walk through that classroom door. (Read Cheryl Oberbeck Burns' story after the following tips for her account of "letting go" when her boys started preschool.) Of course, you can feel more confident of your decision to send your twins to preschool by doing your homework beforehand. Educate yourself about all of the different kinds of preschools that are available. Visit the ones that interest you and make sure you have a full explanation of their policies. Watch how the teachers interact with the children and note how the children respond to their teachers. Talk to other parents in the parking lot about their experiences with the school. Some preschools even have video cameras that allow you to "visit" your children's classroom online from your home or office computer. Following are some tips for helping you and your twins to make the adjustment of entering preschool as painless as possible.

Twins Tips

EASING THE TRANSITION TO PRESCHOOL

- If your twins have always played only with each other, they may have trouble adjusting to having other children in their space. It's important to set up play dates for your twins before they begin preschool. This will get them accustomed to playing—and getting along—with other children. Some twins, on the other hand, may play well with others more quickly because they're more accustomed to playing with a sibling and learning the rules of sharing, cooperation, etc.

- Be aware that if you're hoping to get into a preschool with a very long waiting list, it may be tougher to get in when you're looking for two spots. Be sure to call your desired preschool well before your children are old enough, to find out at what age you can place your kids on the waiting list.

- Paying for preschool for two children can be prohibitive. Find out if the preschool gives a discount for two kids. Perhaps a part-time program would be easier on your finances, as well as on your children's adjustment. Also, if your twins will be there for lunch, find out if the preschool serves food. This will save you the expense of having to provide it and the hassle of packing lunches for your children every morning.

• Find out if your twins will be placed in the same or different classrooms. This may affect your choice of preschools if you're not allowed a choice. (Read the section on schooling in the "Twin Kids" section for additional information on school placement for twins.)

• Ask your prospective preschool about their philosophy and teaching techniques. Some are very academic, while others have very little structure and more play. Select the program that fits your children best. If your twins are very different—perhaps one is mature enough to sit and do lessons, while the other is not—you may want to consider different preschools, or different programs within the same preschool, if available.

• Make sure your preschool teachers take into consideration your twins' relationship. If you feel it's important that your twins be allowed to play and nap together, make sure your preschool is agreeable. If you think your twins need some encouragement to play with others, address that with their teacher(s), too.

• Be aware of your twins' differing needs. One may jump right into preschool without a glance back at you. The other may cling to you for dear life and not want to enter the room. Feel free to give a little extra attention to the child who finds it difficult to separate, but do be firm about saying goodbye. Perhaps the happier child can be enlisted to spend time with her twin when you first leave. Never seek your children's permission to leave or return after you've already left. Most children settle down a few minutes after you've left, or adjust after a week or two when they realize you're always returning to pick them up. A good school has teachers who are sensitive to children's separation anxiety and attempt to get them involved and occupied.

• Allow your twins to each pick out a comfort object to bring to preschool if they're having trouble adjusting, such as a favorite teddy bear or a book. Let their teacher know this helps them feel more comfortable so she doesn't insist they put it away.

• It's important to choose a preschool that meets your children's needs, but make sure it also meets your needs. There are many types of programs, such as Montessori and cooperative.

A cooperative preschool, for instance, requires a lot of parental participation. If you and your husband work many hours or have busy schedules, this may not be the best program for you. Also make sure that the school is licensed, the teachers are qualified, the hours fit your needs, and that the setting is clean and neat. It often helps to get recommendations from other parents. Sometimes the closest preschool isn't necessarily the best one for your family.

Twins Tale
SPRING PARROTS
Cheryl Oberbeck Burns

Before you become a parent, everyone tries to tell you how much you will love your children, but they don't warn you how relentless the love becomes and how lazy days of staring off into space now belong to someone you were long ago, someone you don't feel like anymore. They don't tell you that the years go by like seconds, and no matter how many hours you hold your children and try to memorize every inch of their faces, it still hurts the first morning you ask them, "Are you ready for school?"

My husband and I had decided when our twins were born that we weren't going to buy into the whole "have to go to preschool" fad. After all, we never went to preschool and we turned out okay. It was my pediatrician who convinced me that we should apply to Friends Nursery School. She told me that Friends was a co-op, play based, very nurturing, and, of course, impossible to get into.

Our twin boys, Jack and Chase, were going to be three that summer, and we needed to apply one year ahead to even be considered for admission. So, I set out with the idea of trying to get into Friends. I didn't allow myself to think much past that impossible challenge.

Admissions day was set for the first Saturday morning of October. The school would start taking names via phone until the twenty-five spots were filled. All callers after that would be added to a waiting list.

On the designated morning, I set my alarm and began calling admissions at 8:00 A.M. sharp. I had a landline in one hand and a cell phone in the other. Just like trying to get tickets to a Rolling Stones concert, I was pumped with adrenaline and determined not to miss out. My calls were met with a constant busy signal, but I wasn't going to give up. At 8:10, I finally got through, and our boys' names were added to the list. We filled the last two spots of the 2005 class. I couldn't believe it. I had just won the lottery!

Ten months later, I found myself, along with my husband, sitting in a large meeting room at Friends for the orientation for all new parents. I felt excited and proud to be a part of this renowned school until suddenly it hit me during a teacher presentation on how to label a change of clean clothes for every child: What was I thinking?

I couldn't believe I was really considering leaving my little boys at school without me when they were only three years old. Tears welled up in my eyes. I wondered if the bathrooms were clean. I kept hearing my mom's voice in my head, "Never leave your children until they understand you will be back." I wished my mom were still alive so I could ask for her advice, but she had passed years before ever meeting the boys.

I couldn't ask for her opinion. I had to decide on my own. Were my boys really old enough to fully comprehend that I would be back? And then I came up with a plan. I would call the director in the morning and ask her if she wouldn't mind if I volunteered on both Tuesday and Thursday mornings to help at school. I had already signed up to be a participating parent on Tuesday mornings, but I was sure they could probably use another volunteer on Thursdays. What a great idea!

The next day, Angela, the director, spent an hour on the phone with me. She was very generous and patient. She explained that a small amount of separation was important for the boys and me, and that she would help make sure the boys understood that I would be back to pick them up.

The first day of school, when it was time for parents to depart, Angela offered me a desk in a closed room where I could spend some time watching the boys interact. I could see them, but they could not see me. The boys were interacting, socializing, and having fun within a few short moments. I had said my goodbye moments before and they seemed to understand. I quickly felt comfortable going home.

Truthfully, I did circle around the parking lot a few times before I left, wondering if I should stay just a little longer and hoping that no one would wonder if I had car problems. But it really felt okay to leave—

except for the small nagging feeling that I had forgotten something. I was determined to ignore that feeling, though, especially since I had seen with my own eyes that the parts of me I was leaving behind seemed to be thriving and happy all on their own.

When I got home, I did some laundry and dishes, but I kept my cell phone close. Parents were supposed to be reachable by phone just in case. The phone never rang. The last hour went by quickly. I drove back to school and was so excited to see the boys. I had missed them so much.

At 11:58 A.M. the doors opened, and there were my two happy little boys bursting to throw outstretched arms and painted hands around me. They were all smiles and full of stories about their first morning at school.

Now as I sit here nine months later with kicked-off shoes, pondering that day long ago, I can admire four walls full of artwork: spring parrots, butterflies, Halloween cats, and glittery frogs. I can recount all the seasons, rich with memories and new friends we've made. I have become just another member of a group of parents telling anyone who asks, "Yeah, Friends Nursery School is great!"

Points to Ponder

What type of preschool are you looking into or have you selected? Why is this type optimal for your family?

If your twins have started preschool, how did they each adjust? If they haven't started yet, how do you think your twins will do? What about you . . . how is your separation anxiety?

What benefits will your twins get from attending preschool, such as a head start on academics or increased social skills?

Getting Your Preschoolers to Help Out around the House

As a parent of teenagers who has learned a valuable lesson, I would strongly advise you to get your multiples started on helping out around the house as early as possible. The more it becomes ingrained in their behavior, the easier it will be for you as they get older. Children as young as three can begin to help—and always remember to call it "help," not "work." Little kids love to be parents' helpers and don't even realize that they're doing work when they're granted the "privilege" of doing Mommy's or Daddy's jobs. Start them out, of course, with simple tasks, such as putting silverware on the table for dinner, picking up their toys, giving food to the pets, wiping the table, etc. Gently guide them to do it correctly, but never yell at your kids for doing their jobs "wrong" or not being as good as their sibling(s). Show them the correct way to do the task—even if you have to do it several times and on different occasions. If your children feel like they'll never be able to please you, they'll be reluctant to help out at all. Nancy Johnson has a great system for enlisting her triplets' help with the laundry.

Twins Tips
MAKING LAUNDRY A FAMILY AFFAIR
Nancy Johnson

Our family has a great system for keeping the house organized and getting the kids to help. Each child has a small plastic basket inside his or her closet that serves as a hamper. The children bring their baskets to the laundry room in the morning after collecting stray socks and other clothes off their bedroom floor. They sort their dirty laundry into a three-bin sorter for whites, mediums, and darks. Then, they bring the little baskets back into their rooms.

My kids have been sorting their own dirty laundry since they were around three years old. They don't always get the sorting right, but the idea is there and I don't have to run all over the house searching under beds for dirty clothes! They even help me wash, dry, and fold their clothes now (which has cut down on the four or five outfits a day they were wearing!).

Points to Ponder

In what ways do your multiples help out around the house?

What does it take, if anything, to motivate your kids to help with chores?

What are the advantages of assigning jobs to kids at an early age?

A Final Word

What's the best piece of advice I can offer for raising toddler twins? *Just love them.* So many parents take for granted the incredible gift they've been given in the form of their children. We are so blessed! So, the next time your toddlers drive you to the brink of insanity, take a deep breath and remember just how much you love them. Look at each of their little features and marvel at their perfection. Be awed by how smart and clever and ingenious they are (even when they're applying these traits to figuring out how to escape their bedroom!). It's difficult to stay mad for long when you're in love. Remember why you wanted these children and think of how full and rich your life is now that they're here. Sure, it's chaotic, but someday you're going to miss those tiny little socks on the floor. And, yes, you might even fondly remember Elmo's squeaky voice or Barney's dopey laugh. The days when your little ones are all tucked into their beds with their favorite stuffed animals and wearing their footed pajamas will soon be past.

Trust me, years from now, it won't be the tantrums you'll remember; it will be the sloppy kisses. It won't be the hits. It will be the hugs. It won't be "No!" It will be "Mama" and that sweet little breath in your face. So, remember to love them. They are precious, indeed.

Twins Tale

LOVING TWINS
John C. Flewellen

Twins are wonderful,
Twins are neat,
Twins are born
With four little feet.

Twins make you laugh,
And make you cry.
Always curious,
Always asking why.

Then they start growing,
Big girls, big boys.
They still are wonderful
And still want toys.

Identical twins,
That's what I got.
Over the years
They have fought.

We love our twins,
And will forever.
They are in our prayers,
Until the twelfth of never.

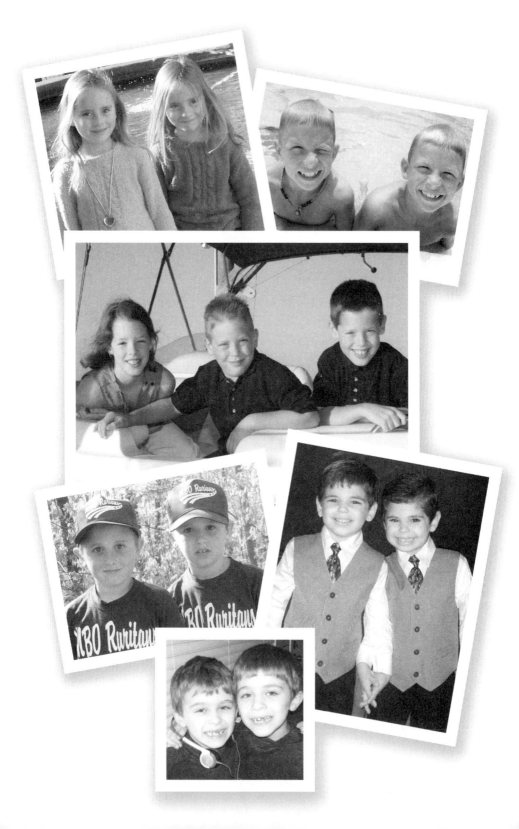

Part 3

Twin Kids
(Ages 5–11)

I have very fond memories of the elementary school years with my singleton children (now teens). Now that you're finally getting some sleep, I think you'll especially treasure these years with your twins, too. After many challenges along the way, they've emerged at last from the infant and toddler years and are now full-fledged kids ready for every experience you can offer! There are many things to love about these years. Family vacations are now more fun and less work. Your twins still want to be in your company, and yet don't insist you entertain them every minute. They're developing many different interests, from sports to dance, from dolls to dinosaurs, from clothes to games, etc. You don't have to haul a super-sized diaper bag or stroller along every time you need to run an errand. Your twins can play independently while you actually read a book for pleasure or cook a nice meal. You will understand their homework (before they hit calculus), and they're not humiliated if you volunteer to be the room parent or chaperone a field trip. Yes, twin kids are great!

Of course, despite this glorious picture I've painted, there are challenges during these years. Like any siblings, your twins may engage in competition or even all-out battles! They're still going to act up in school and at the grocery store. They'll be adjusting each year to a new classroom and friends—with or without each other. And you'll see their separate personalities emerge even more as opportunities arise for exploring individual interests. You might be running one to the soccer field, while your spouse is running the other to the basketball court. One may come home in tears every night as she adjusts to a new classroom, while the other easily fits in with others her age. You'll constantly be trying to balance the needs of two children (plus any others you may be raising), and the issues are going to be different from those you've encountered before.

So, cherish these very memorable years with your twins. Before you know it, they'll be out of elementary school, and a new set of challenges will await them—and you!

It's Time for School!
Should Your Twins Be Placed
Together or in Separate Classrooms?

When your twins are ready to start school, the big question is always whether they will be better off in the same class or different classes (assuming there is more than one class in their grade level at that school). First of all, you should know that you may not have a choice! Some schools require that twins be placed in separate classrooms. If you'd prefer that your twins be in the same class, you'll want to do your research well before it's time for the kids to start school. You may choose to move your children to a school that is more willing to work with your requests, or you may wish to explore your options to fight the policy, as did Wendy M. Haavisto of Minnesota. When her boy/girl twins were forced into separate classes at the start of first grade, she took her fight all the way to the state legislature, where a bill was signed into law on May 5, 2005, giving parents of multiples the right to choose whether their children are placed in the same or different classrooms. Parents in many other states are now pushing for similar laws.

With that in mind, and assuming you *do* have a choice, you should know that there are advantages and disadvantages to both options.

Advantages of Placing Twins in Different Classrooms

- Your children are more likely to be judged as individuals rather than as a unit. Comparisons between the two will be avoided.
- If your twins tend to play only with each other, having them in different classrooms might help them to make new friends and be more sociable.
- Your twins will be less distracted by each other and better able to focus on their work.
- They'll have to do their own homework, as it is likely to be different. One can't rely on the other to do the work or supply the answers.
- If one twin lives in the shadow of the other, this may allow the shyer, less confident child to shine.

Advantages of Placing Twins in the Same Classroom

- Your children will experience equal instructional quality. One won't get the "bad teacher," while the other benefits from one who's better qualified.
- It will be easier to help them with homework when they have the same assignments, and they can help each other as well.
- It will be easier for you to participate in the classroom when you're not stretched between two different classrooms (especially if you also have other children in other classes).
- As starting school can be an adjustment for any child, having a brother or sister in the classroom can make the adjustment less traumatic.
- They'll have each other's ears in the classroom. If one misses

the details of an assignment, the other may hear it and repeat it at home.

If you feel your twins would do better together, but your school has a strict policy of separate classrooms—and you don't feel you have the resources to fight it or move—consider taking a "wait and see policy." Tell your twins to give separation a try for a certain period of time, say six months, to see how things go. Some families are pleasantly surprised at how well their twins adjust to separate classrooms after a period of time. Cindy Ferraino's twins, Lyndsey and Erika, were separated in kindergarten, while Sherry St. James's boy/girl twins stayed together until separating in second grade. Both mothers had reservations about separating their twins at first, but ultimately found their decision to be the best for their twins.

Twins Tale
TWIN POWER!
Cindy Ferraino

My seven-year-old identical twins, Lyndsey and Erika, have been in separate classrooms since kindergarten. This has worked out very well for them. That first year, the two-and-a-half-hour program gave our girls the opportunity to meet new friends and share in some wonderful experiences without affecting their strong twin bond. Our decision to separate was beneficial, and we looked forward to that year when they would be in first grade. Again, the twins have adjusted well. As for Mom and Dad, well, we are still coping.

On one occasion, both teachers assigned the same homework. I thought this might be a great idea. With a single assignment, surely we could fly through homework time! But having the same homework gave Lyndsey another thought about what an advantage it would be to share a classroom with Erika.

"Mommy," she explained, "we could help each other out with homework, and you could take a break!"

Such a sweet child, I thought sarcastically. *Always thinking of me. Okay, what does she really mean?*

Erika offered up an explanation. "Lyndsey could do half the homework, and I could do the other!"

Ah, I should have known. Lyndsey and Erika had harnessed their "twin power" to pull a fast one over on Mommy! Carefully, I explained that even though Mommy could use a break once in a while, they still needed to do their homework alone. Needless to say, Lyndsey and Erika were not pleased with my reply.

I began to pray for different homework from their teachers. Ever since my plea, we have not gotten the same homework!

Twins Tale

TO SPLIT OR NOT TO SPLIT
Sherry St. James

Be careful what you wish for, my mother would always say. *You just might get it.* She was right. For as long as I could remember, I wanted to be the mother of twins. When I was thirty-two, I got my wish. I can still hear the doctor's voice, "Congratulations! It's a girl . . . and a boy!" Perfect! Just like I always wanted.

From the time my twins were born, I was one of those moms who didn't mind the novelty of having multiples. I loved it. Most of the questions I enjoyed. My twins are connected in a way above and beyond that of typical siblings, making their "twinness" very special. But, as they approached school age, the questions changed. Increasingly often I was asked when, not normally *if*, but *when* I would split them up. The idea of ever splitting them up hadn't crossed my mind. I was a mother of *twins*, after all, not one daughter and one son who happened to be born at the same time.

There was a time when the thought of separating twins in school, or any time before adulthood for that matter, was taboo. Twins were thought to be uniquely bonded and so kept together. That time has passed. Twins are now expected to grow up separately and function independently. Today the thought is not so much *if* twins should be separated, but *when*.

But how could I separate them? I loved everything about being a twin mom, even the exhausting parts, like breastfeeding twins on two very different schedules. I think because they were so special, I felt special as well. Surely my twins didn't need to be split up.

I've always been interested to hear about the varying degrees of twin bonding. Some twins are competitive, some grow apart intellectually or academically, and some twins, even identical twins, do not share much of a bond at all. A few twins even seem to have problems with each other and are adamant about their individuality. But then there are those who seem to maintain a connection so precious, so amazing, and so strong that the thought of them separating is something anyone who knows them cannot fathom. My twins are like this. They have a bond that touches everyone who knows them.

When one is afraid, the other is brave. When one is hurt, the other comes to the rescue. They share sadness. They share joy. They even share the same goofy sense of humor.

Just the other day, my daughter accidentally shut the car door on her twin brother's foot. He shrieked, but he wasn't hurt. She felt so bad about it that she began to cry while apologizing profusely. He was so moved by her heartfelt apology that he began to cry with her while assuring her he was okay. They held each other and cried and comforted each other so lovingly that I began to cry! Then, we all ended up laughing hysterically. That's just how it is with my twins. They are amazing to be around. I feel so blessed to be their mother.

When I sent them to preschool two days a week, I didn't even consider separating them—and neither did their preschool teachers. They sat at the same table and next to each other in the circle, played together at recess, and rested side by side during quiet time. At school as at home, they preferred to spend most of their time together. Their teachers, like me, adored their special bond.

When kindergarten came, I kept them together and didn't give it a second thought. My twins had no difficulties sharing the same classroom even though they were so close. They regularly walked into school hand in hand, and often held hands on the way out to recess and to music or gym. It was precious. They sat at different tables and worked in different groups, but their teacher said they always needed to sit in such a way that they could see each other. All their teachers respected that. As long as one twin knew where the other one was, they functioned effectively and independently. I thought this was sweet.

Then we were faced with the big decision: Do we split them up in first grade? They both were advancing academically at virtually the same pace. They maintained separate friendships, yet played together as often as they played apart. There seemed to be no reason to split them up. I loved being the mother of these precious twins, together in one classroom, but of course, I wanted what was best for them. Then I asked them what they wanted—a seemingly simple idea at the time.

Apparently, the thought of separating had never, ever crossed their young minds. They completely fell apart at the mere idea! They cried and panicked and held on to each other as if there were no tomorrow. Had I projected my own feelings of staying together on to them? Or was their bond really this incredible? Of course, I dropped the idea of separation after such a display. At this point, I don't think I was ready to see them separated yet either, so I didn't push.

After much discussion with their kindergarten teacher, we decided to keep the twins together for first grade and to reevaluate for second grade. We had no real reason to split them up. They functioned independently, and quite honestly, that bond was so obvious and so endearing that I think we just couldn't bring ourselves to interfere with it. I know I couldn't do it. Last and yes least, it was much more convenient for me to have them in the same classroom. Plus, I continued to love the experience of being the mother of these amazingly close twins who shared everything, even a classroom.

Keeping my twins together for first grade proved to be a success. They grew more independent, and while they continued to keep tabs on each other, they grew to rely on each other less and less. One substitute teacher told me she never would have guessed they were even related had a classmate not mentioned it to her. They each became more autonomous because their teacher was careful to always treat them as individuals. At the same time, she completely respected their bond, and even nurtured it. Fortunately for us, this teacher was amazing—above and beyond anyone we could have hoped for. She worked not only on my twins, but on me as well.

I remember one particular conference when she began with, "Let's talk about this separation anxiety."

"Whose?" I asked. "His or hers?"

"Yours," she lovingly replied. Then we laughed until we cried. I suppose the mother of twins must deal with her own separation issues as well.

Soon enough, we were faced with that same decision again: to split or not to split. This time we had a slightly different situation. My twins were older, and at this school, the second grade teachers team-teach in an open setting. Although I still saw no need to split up my twins, this seemed to be the perfect opportunity to separate them very gently and gradually, just to see how it goes—for all of us. We discussed the importance of their individuality, as well as the need to foster their special bond. The teachers understood and agreed to make the effort necessary to take special care of my twins—and their mom.

The grownups all agreed, but of course, we still had to convince my twins. At first I was met with opposition. Not adamant—no clinging, no tears—but neither twin seemed willing to separate. My son was more open to the idea, but sensing his sister's apprehension, he quickly renounced it. I was determined, this time, not to let my emotions show. Was I ready to give up the novelty of being the mother of these remarkable twins in the same class? No. But this wasn't about me. Fairly certain that we would regret this missed opportunity, I lovingly persuaded them (and myself) to at least give it a try. Once my daughter agreed, my son was quick to follow.

They were ready, not because they had been separated before, but because they had been allowed to grow individually together.

I believe there is no easy answer to the twin separation issue—not for the twins or the mothers of twins. As adults, we need to remember that being a twin, especially a connected, bonded twin, is indeed a very important part of the very autonomy we wish to encourage. There is no hurry. Separation will happen naturally, when they are ready.

Good teachers who understand and respect the tricky situation surrounding being a bonded twin are a must. And for me, dealing with my own separation anxiety made helping my twins deal with theirs much easier. Separating twins in school is inevitable, truly a matter of *when*, not *if*.

What we must remember is that there is no rush and that separation doesn't make them any less twins—or their mother any less the mother of twins.

Points to Ponder

What is your school's policy, if it has one, about twin placement in classrooms? Do you like or dislike this policy? If you dislike it, do you plan to fight it, move to another district, or just put up with it?

If your twins haven't started school yet, do you think they'll do better in the same or different classrooms? Why?

If your twins do attend school now, are they in the same or different classrooms? How has this worked out for your family?

Twins Tips

HANDLING HOMEWORK WITHOUT "MULTIPLE" HASSLES!

- With twins, especially if they're in different classrooms, it's more difficult for you to keep track of their assignments, class trips, teacher requests, etc. Teach your children at an early age to empty their backpacks as soon as they get home to give you any announcements or papers distributed by the teacher. Also, remind them to write down their assignments and to bring home all the books they need to do their homework.

- Give each twin her own workspace. If twins sit together at the same table, they may get distracted easily. If they have the same homework, sitting together makes it too tempting for them to do their homework together or to copy each other. Even if they have different homework, they may tend to interrupt each other with questions and comments about their day.

- Be conscious of each child's individual need for relaxation. Some twins need a little unwinding time when they get home before starting their homework. Others might be able to jump right into their homework to get it over with. Let each twin do as he wishes, but stick to a schedule. If one wants to have a snack first, agree that snack time will last for a half-hour, and then it's time for homework. If the other child gets started on his homework right away, remind him that it's important to be quiet if he finishes his homework before his brother does.

- When your twins come home from school, they're often eager to share news about their day and may compete to give you the latest news first or to come up with the best story. It's important to set guidelines. Let your twins take turns giving their news, and don't allow one child to interrupt the other with his or her own version of a story or to "one up" the other. Teach your twins to listen respectfully to each other's stories and to wait for their turn. If one or both are upset about something, make sure to schedule some private, one-on-one time with the troubled child to give your full attention to the matter.

- Let your twins pick out different backpacks, lunch bags, notebooks, and folders. It often helps to have each child pick a particular color or theme. This makes it easy to find each child's things and none of you will get mixed up.

- Never compare your twins' skills. If one masters multiplication tables in a week, but the other is still struggling, never remind the struggler that her twin learned them faster. And don't allow your twins to compete with each other. If one says to the other, "You're so stupid. Anyone knows that six times eight equals forty-eight," remind him how he would feel if his twin teased him about something he wasn't good at. Teach them to put themselves in each other's shoes when it comes to teasing and name-calling. And let them know that learning new things at different paces is normal.

- Mornings can be chaotic with multiples, so have your twins get all of their school things ready the night before. Put all completed homework in backpacks and have them at the door or in the car. Set out clothes for the next day. Place bowls and cereal on the counter for breakfast the next morning. The more organized you are the night before, the less chaos you'll experience the next morning.

Points to Ponder

Do your twins do their homework together or separately? How has this worked out?

What techniques do you employ for getting your twins to do their homework?

How do you teach your twins to be organized when it comes to doing homework and getting ready for school?

Do you find that your twins compete with each other when it comes to class assignments? How do you curb this rivalry?

Encouraging Twins to Play with Others

Is it wrong for twins to want to be together? Of course not! The bond between twins is beautiful, and most parents melt at the sight of their twins holding hands or looking out for one another. This is wonderful and a real benefit for your children, who always have the loving support of their sibling. However, your twins must also grow up in the real world and learn to interact with other people. If one of the goals of raising children is to prepare them for adulthood and reality, then they need to be encouraged to develop close relationships with others.

One of the ways to facilitate getting your children to know other children is to treat your multiples as individuals and to encourage them to pursue separate interests. If one child likes soccer and the other would rather play baseball, never make them choose one or the other. Allow them to take different classes or to join separate teams—even if it means more running around for you and your partner. This is beneficial because it will help your twins make more friends with similar interests. And, by being in social situations apart from each other, they're more likely to be seen as individuals rather than as part of a set. Joining a sports team also puts children in situations where they must cooperate with others—a valuable social skill—although twins already have an advantage in this, as they've been learning to cooperate with each other all their lives!

Give your twins many opportunities to develop separate friendships. You might have Grandma pick up one for an outing while the other has a friend over. (Then switch places the next week.) Of course, if your twins are in separate classrooms, this may also encourage them to play with other children. If your multiples are in the same classroom, talk to their teacher to see if they are playing only with each other. If so, develop strategies with their teacher that will encourage your kids to play with others. Perhaps the teacher can place them at separate tables or on different relay teams. If children are asked to pick partners for school projects, they should be encouraged to pick a child other than their twin.

If one child is invited to an outing with a friend and the other isn't, don't necessarily jump in to ask that both children be allowed to attend, even if the uninvited child is upset. Use this as an opportunity to spend some one-on-one time with the twin who is staying home, or encourage this child to have her own friend over to the house. If your twins are close, reassure them that having separate friends doesn't mean that they have to give up their relationship with one another. One twin may feel more insecure than the other about "losing" her brother or sister. Let this child know that she will always have her twin, and that making friends is a natural part of growing up.

Developing social skills is an important part of the school years for all children. But this can be especially challenging for twins because they're accustomed to having their very own playmate at hand. With a bit of encouragement, your multiples can reap the benefits of having a best friend (their twin) by their side, as well as many other friends in the outside world.

Points to Ponder

Are your twins best friends? What are the benefits and drawbacks of this relationship?

Do your twins have any separate interests? How can you encourage them to develop or pursue different activities?

Do your twins socialize with other children and pursue friendships? What ideas do you have for encouraging them to make friends with others?

Twins Trivia

DO IDENTICAL TWINS HAVE THE SAME FINGERPRINTS?

You might be surprised to learn that identical twins are not identical in every way. It's not clear why, but they have different fingerprints! This often comes in handy when parents take their identical twins home from the hospital and remove their hospital bracelets. If they can't tell the twins apart, they can be fingerprinted again and matched with the prints taken at the hospital. I read a true story once about twin baby girls who lost their hospital bracelets. It seemed that their older brother was very good at telling them apart, so the parents let the brother identify the twins for them. About twelve years later, they were fingerprinted and found that the brother had been wrong! After being called by the "wrong" names for so many years, the twins had, of course, become accustomed to them, so they chose to correct their birth certificates rather than change their names.

Intriguing Twins
TIA AND TAMERA MOWRY

Tia and Tamera Mowry were born on July 6, 1978, to military parents stationed in Gelhausen, Germany. Because of their parents' careers, the identical twins moved around quite a bit, including stints in Texas and Honolulu. The girls didn't mind this too much since there were always plenty of other kids around, but sometimes it was tough to adjust to changing schools and friends so frequently. But being twins turned out to be a plus with this type of lifestyle since they always had each other! The girls grew very close and did everything together, but they also wanted to be known as individuals and would correct people who called them merely "the twins."

When they lived in Texas, Tamera began to compete in pageants. Tia didn't want to participate at first, but when she saw how successful her sister was, she changed her mind. Soon they both began winning pageants and talent shows. When Tia and Tamera were twelve, they decided they wanted to become actresses, and they begged their parents to move to California. Their mother told them that they would go there for a month, and if they managed to get an acting job during that time, they would move there. It took almost the whole month, but the girls finally got a job doing a commercial for an automobile company, so the family moved to Los Angeles in 1990.

While attending high school, the twins continued to audition for small roles and commercials, and achieved some success. During this time, their little brother, Tahj, landed a recurring role on the hit TV show *Full House*. Through this connection, the twins met a woman named Irene Dreayer at de Passe Entertainment, and she dreamed up the idea for a show just for the twins called *Sister Sister*. The show became an overwhelming success!

The twins are out of college now, and continue to act and do charitable work. Tia and Tamera are extremely talented twins!

Planning Birthday Parties for the School-Age Set

You can get away with joint gifts and cakes when twins are babies and toddlers, but once they reach school age, personal preferences and individual treatment should be given respect. Twins learn to accept that they have to share a birthday (unless one was born before midnight and the other after!), but they still want to be treated like other kids and have their own special day—one that's tailored just for them!

Twins Tips
MAKING BIRTHDAYS SPECIAL FOR YOUR MULTIPLES

- You can probably get away with a joint party, but separate cakes, candles, and birthday songs are a must. Sing "Happy Birthday" to each child individually (you can alternate years on who goes first!), and let them each select their favorite kind of cake. (You can always make the cakes smaller if you're concerned about having too much, or make cupcakes and let each twin choose the flavor and decorations for half.) Each child deserves the chance to be in the limelight alone, at least for a few minutes.

- Many parents, relatives, and friends of twins wonder if it's okay to give a joint gift. Let's put it this way: Just because twins happen to share a birthday doesn't mean they should share a gift. If you had a child with a birthday in April and another child with a birthday in June, would your June birthday child be happy if you told him that his gift was the other half of what his brother received in April? Of course not! Regardless of when their birthdays fall, kids want their own stuff. Twins are just as possessive as other kids! There are certainly exceptions, as in the case of major items like swing sets, but in general twins should get their own gifts—preferably those that express their personalities. If one twin likes dolls and the other prefers games, don't get them both dolls. It's okay to get each twin something totally different, unless they specifically ask for the same thing. The goal is to make your twins feel special by recognizing that their own personal interests are valid. Giving a joint gift and forcing the twins to share does not reflect a concern for their individuality. So, encourage guests to bring separate gifts. You might want to consider sending two invitations—one from each child. Or, you can write a little hint on the invitation: "Mary loves Barbies; Julie enjoys soccer!"

- Let each child choose her own guests. Of course, cousins and other family members will be joint guests, but make sure that each twin has a few special friends included just for him or her, even if the guest is not acquainted with both children. (This may happen especially if your twins are in different classrooms.)

- Again, give your twins a lot of individual choice. Let them each select their own invitations, games to play, birthday outfits, decorations, etc. Don't impose a theme on them that they don't both like just because you think it's cute or convenient for twins. If your daughter loves Dora the Explorer and your son loves Spider-Man, don't hesitate to combine them at the party. The guests won't mind a bit!

- Take a picture of every guest with each twin alone, holding his or her gift from the recipient. (If the guest didn't get the hint and gives a joint gift anyway, you'll need to include both twins in the picture.) If you decide to have your children open gifts after the party, include the wrapped gift in the picture. When the party's over, each twin can personalize the picture with a thank you message and signature, which can be mailed to the party guest. Each twin should write his or her own thank you notes. Separate gifts require separate notes!

- Let each twin select his or her own party favors for guests. (Certainly, no guest will complain about getting two party favors!) Hit a dollar store to cut down on expenses, or get creative and make your own small gifts.

- Don't necessarily rule out having separate parties if your twins really want them. Offer them the choice of one bigger party, or allow two smaller ones. For instance, each child can have two to three other children over on separate nights for a sleepover. A party at home or the park is much less expensive than at a bowling alley or roller rink, where there's often a ten kid minimum. Listen to your twins' preferences if they're reasonable. Mary Reeves came up with the following idea that allowed each of her twins to have a special day of her own: "Our identical twin girls share pretty much everything. We wanted to do something for their seventh birthdays that would allow each of them to feel really special. We chose the weekend prior to their birthday. Each got to plan their own day that would include two meals at home, one meal out, and an activity she wanted to do that day. Once they made their plans, Mommy made a sign for each that was titled "Name's Special Day" and listed the plans for that day. Each ended up choosing a special breakfast at home, a favorite restaurant for lunch, an afternoon activity, and a homemade dinner at home. The whole weekend was a lot of fun."

And what should be done if one twin is invited to someone else's birthday party and the other isn't? First, gauge the excluded twin's level of upset. Some children are mature enough to understand that they might not get to go to this party but will be invited to another. This is especially true of boy/girl twins. Usually, if you explain that "Mandy is going to an all-girls party," then Joseph understands and doesn't feel he's missing out. Even with singleton children, it's a good lesson to learn that they won't be the recipient of every invitation. In some cases, especially if twins are in different classes at school, a parent may not realize that the invited child is a twin. A discreet call to the child's parent may rectify the situation and get the other child invited without realizing he or she was excluded. The other alternative is to plan something special with the excluded twin. Say to your child, "Devon is going to a birthday party this afternoon, so you and I get to go to the movies! We'll have a special day of our own." Let your child know that you're looking forward to spending some time alone together.

Twins Tale

TWINS: PARTY OF TWO
Sherry St. James

One birthday + two birthday kids = annual dilemma. As if kids' birthday parties weren't complicated enough, mothers of twins face a unique birthday party predicament year after year. Shared party or separate parties? Simultaneous parties or staggered parties? Shared day or separate days? Trying to choose and plan can make a twin mom want to skip the party altogether! Most importantly, we must figure out our own expectations of the party: what we want it to be and why.

The first twin birthday is easy. The babies are only one year old, after all, and they have no idea what is going on. Invite some family, mash the fingers in the cake and the cake on the face, snap a few pictures, and you have yourself the cutest party of the year. Ten minutes of oohs and aahs, let Grandma rinse the kids in the shower, a couple more pictures, and that party is a big success! We want the whole world to celebrate the shared birthday of these precious twins, and we are proud when they do.

The second party is also pretty easy. Think of the endless theme possibilities of your two kids turning two! My duo had their Noah's Ark theme party at 2:02 P.M. on 02/02/2000. It was a predictable, double everything party—and a huge success. I have, you guessed it, two pages of pictures of this pair from this fun day. Our family and friends still talk about that day of double trouble. We hoped for fun and happy memories, still playing up the twinness, and this party still provides entertainment for all.

Now, birthday party number three is where things begin to get complicated. The kids know what a birthday is *and* what a party is. They have probably even been to a few, and they may want one of their own. Alone. In our case, my boy/girl twins turned three on the third of February, so we had to do something special for this "golden birthday" (you know, five on the fifth, ten on the tenth—we all have one by the time we are thirty-one, even though many of us overlook it). I told them that if they shared the party, it could be big and really something special. They liked that idea, so we rented out a gymnastics academy at three o'clock on the third for three hours and had the time of our thirty-something lives! The kids had a great time, too. The idea was all for fun and fun for all.

So far so good.

Then the dreaded day came in early January, when my twin son announced he wanted a cowboy party for their fourth birthday. My twin daughter, dressed in pink frills and covered with glitter, completely balked at this idea. She was determined to have a princess party. Now I had a problem. Both great ideas, but not a compromise in sight. I realized it was time to make the break. I wanted to give them what they asked for.

We sent out pink invitations to all the girls, and they graced the party in dress-up costumes and enjoyed makeovers, manicures, and a royal tea party. All the female friends and relatives came to the princess party, and it was a lot of fun.

We sent rodeo invites to all the boys, and they showed up in cowboy attire and practiced sheriff shootouts with cap guns and imaginary calf roping. All the male friends and relatives came to the cowboy party, and it was a lot of fun . . . or so I heard. I can't say firsthand because *I* was at the princess party. My husband donned his cowboy hat over at the O.K. Corral and assured me it was a boot-scootin' good time.

For the guests' convenience, we scheduled these parties in two nearby locations at the same time. I didn't consider this a problem until my daughter asked why she didn't get to go to her twin brother's party, and he asked the same of hers. Then I realized that all of us missed one of their parties. This may not be a problem for some, but in our house we don't like to miss each other's parties! While the twins had a great time, they missed not having each other at their parties, and quite frankly, I was sad that I missed my son's party. To make matters worse, no one remembered a camera, and it wasn't like I could go back and take more pictures! I wanted to give them their way, and the parties were fun, but only being able to go to one was a problem for many of us—most importantly, the birthday twins themselves.

For birthday number five, they were back together with a small, after-school party at home with just a few guests and grandparents. The idea was to keep things simple and to keep them together. That went well, for me at least, but it seemed a bit low key for the party pair. So for the next year, we decided to let them plan their own parties.

After careful thought, the twins decided to share their sixth birthday party at a kids' pizza and game place, but they wanted different themed cakes and plates on two tables side by side. This was a great solution, and most of the girls naturally gathered around my daughter and her Hello Kitty favors, while the boys gravitated to the Spider-Man stuff. In the past, we had always requested *no gifts*, much to my children's chagrin, but at this party, we inadvertently overlooked this little tidbit of information. While my twins were thrilled with all the plastic plunder, I felt bad that the parents all had to bring two gifts. We wanted all the kids to have fun, but we didn't consider the twofold expense for the parents this time.

For party number seven, we encountered a new twist. *He* wanted the children's place with the kid-sized hamster tubes. *She* wanted a sleepover. And *neither* wanted to miss the other's party. *I* wanted to try a new approach. To accomplish this, we had two parties at different times on the same day. His friends were invited to the afternoon game place party, and she and one other girl got to go. Her friends were invited to the sleepover later that night, and he got to have one boy spend the night as well. This was a fabulous compromise on everyone's part. Each twin got to feel special and solo in the spotlight, yet neither sibling missed out on the other's party. Parents who brought gifts only provided one. Everyone who wanted to could go to both parties. This new approach was a big success.

Birthday parties can be a trick to pull off, and twin parties present even more of a challenge. Next year, my twins will turn eight, and I have no idea what they will want. I know I want something collectively simple that all can enjoy. Now that we have tried so many different party plans, I am confident that whatever we choose, we will find an approach that can work for everyone.

Points to Ponder

What has been your most memorable birthday party for your twins? Did you hold a joint party or separate parties? What are your plans for the next birthday?

How do you encourage guests to bring separate gifts? Do your twins mind getting joint gifts, or do they prefer separate ones?

Do you have any birthday traditions that help each twin feel special?

The Importance of Family Traditions

Birthdays are a great time to institute family traditions. Perhaps you have a special birthday plate (or two) for your multiples on which to place their cake! Some families sing a silly song or make a special treat reserved for this day. But birthdays aren't the only times to institute family traditions. Holidays are wonderful occasions to practice rituals that your extended family may have been performing for generations. This is a good time to teach lasting values to your twins, such as the importance of family, giving to others, the practice of faith, love for God, or respect for one's country. And, of course, traditions also allow us to have fun! They make us feel good and give us something to look forward to. They may be as simple as having popcorn and a movie every Friday night. Or, they might be as elaborate as having a Christmas light display that rivals Clark Griswold's in the *Christmas Vacation* movie. Twins are especially conscious of identity issues, and traditions are helpful in giving your children a sense of belonging and a place in the family. Give each of your multiples a special privilege of their choice when it comes to family traditions. For example, one child may wish to say the prayer at Christmas dinner, while the other wants to read the nativity story. Emphasize that each role is an extremely valuable part of the holiday ritual. The yearly—or even weekly—practice of traditions gives children good memories that they will cherish for a lifetime. Indeed, I guarantee that the Reeves twins will be talking for the rest of their lives about Tooth Fairy Bob's visit to their house!

Twins Tale

TOOTH FAIRY BOB STRIKES AGAIN
Mary Reeves

Melony, one of our twin daughters, lost a tooth at school. When she got home, she showed it to Daddy and then left it on the kitchen island counter in a small, lidless tooth-shaped container that the school nurse had given her. I didn't realize it was there when I proceeded to prepare our dinner. After the meal, I suddenly heard Melony crying. Her tooth was gone! The container was still upright on the counter, but where in the world had the tiny tooth gone? We began to search all over, and I even swept the floor and checked the dustpan. Daddy and I kept reassuring Melony that the tooth fairy would still visit that night, even if we didn't find the tooth, but she was so upset that Daddy decided to sneak a dollar under her pillow while we were searching. We told her that maybe the tooth fairy had snuck in while the girls had been jamming to "Bohemian Rhapsody" with Daddy as Mommy was cleaning up from dinner. Daddy said that perhaps "Tooth Fairy Bob" (he had convinced the girls there are boy fairies as well as girl fairies) had such a busy night ahead that he needed to take care of some teeth early. Melony was adamant, though, that it couldn't have happened that way at all! Nevertheless, Daddy convinced her to go to her room and search just in case. Because we have special tooth pillows that we had put on the nightstand when Melony lost her first tooth, she didn't automatically think to check her real pillow on her bed. Daddy somehow got her to look there, and he said the expression on her face was absolutely price-less when she discovered the dollar underneath! She came running out to show me, dancing around and totally in awe that Tooth Fairy Bob could have snuck in while we were all awake! Later, as we were kissing her goodnight, she said it was the best day of her whole life!

Points to Ponder

What beloved traditions did you and your spouse practice when you were children?

What rituals does your family practice frequently, such as a pizza night or singing a special goodnight song?

What annual holiday traditions does your family especially look forward to?

Twins Trivia

DO TWINS SKIP A GENERATION?

There is no scientific proof that giving birth to twins skips a generation. Of course, it sometimes happens, but twins can just as easily be conceived in every generation of a family, or once and never again! However, women in a particular family can have a genetic predisposition for producing more than one egg during a menstrual cycle, therefore making them more likely to conceive twins. This is why it sometimes seems that twins run in the family. Note that since these twins are the result of multiple eggs being fertilized, this genetic component only holds true for fraternal twins.

Are You Suffering from Memory Loss?

If you're like me, you frequently enter a room to retrieve something and forget what you wanted. Or, you spy someone you know in the grocery store but can't for the life of you remember her name. Or, perhaps you emerge from the store to find that you can't remember where you parked your car. If you find this happening to you more frequently, you're not alone. Being the parent of twins (and perhaps other children) is certainly a stressor and a sleep depriver, which can play havoc with your brain. But, sorry to say, this also goes with the territory when you enter middle age. Scientists aren't sure why—perhaps we begin to lose brain cells, or perhaps our brain cells just don't communicate as well as they used to—but chances are slim that you're suffering from Alzheimer's, as you've probably feared. Memory loss is most likely caused by age and stress. And parents of multiples are masters at multi-tasking, which tends to clutter the brain. That's why it's helpful to keep a very accurate calendar and a to-do list (if you could only remember to check it . . . after you find it!). At my house, I instruct my kids to write any food they use up or finish on the grocery list posted on the refrigerator because I know

I'm not going to remember when one of them says, "Mom, we're out of milk!" And in the drawer I keep a calendar that I check several times a day, on which I've written every single activity I must attend, even if it's a regular event. You might want to keep a notepad in your purse in case you remember something while you're out that you need to do later. Some people even leave themselves messages on their cell phones or carry small voice recorders. When you write things down, you won't be stressed about forgetting them. (Of course, if your memory loss seems to get worse with time and even list-making doesn't seem to help, please see your doctor to be checked out.) Most of all, and I know it's difficult, try to get plenty of rest, nutrition, and exercise, and manage your stress. All of these things are good for the brain and allow you to achieve optimum mental functionality—something you certainly need when you're running after multiples!

Twins Tale
CONFESSIONS OF A MUDDLE-AGED MOM OF MULTIPLES
Lisa Crystal

Leopard-spotted slippers will forever remind me of things forgotten. One bright December day, I purchased a pair for Christmas for my jungle crazed eleven-year-old, Nina. After she went to bed that night, I showed them to my husband, Mark. Then I put them away.

On the night of December 23rd, Mark and I were knee deep in wrapping paper, getting a head start on the Christmas Eve packaging marathon. I'd prepared most of the goodies for our five-year-old twin boys, but I couldn't find my daughter's slippers. In a panic, I searched all the usual hiding places, to no avail. "I did show them to you, right?" I asked Mark. He nodded thoughtfully, brow furrowed. I tried to conjure an image of what I did after I showed them to him without success. I must have thrown them away with the packaging from the other items I had purchased that day. I resolved to return to the discount store the next day and find another pair.

But, on the day before Christmas, the girls' slipper rack was stripped bare, save for a pink fuzzy variety. I phoned Mark at his downtown office. Surely somewhere in the city he could locate a pair of leopard slippers. Oddly, he found some at a sporting goods store, albeit at more than double the cost of the original pair from our suburban discounter. No matter—our girl would have her slippers come Christmas morning.

And the next day Nina was indeed thrilled when she opened her gift, and immediately put them on. She was less excited when, a half-hour later, she opened the last package under the tree and pulled out . . . leopard-spotted slippers! From the discount store. She and Mark looked at me quizzically, and I suddenly recalled thinking how smart it would be to wrap some gifts and stick them under the tree as I purchased them. Clearly that plan had lasted for only one gift. More troubling was that I had absolutely no recollection of actually boxing up the slippers and tucking them under the tree. An action I had performed only three weeks ago had vanished from my memory—if it had ever been there at all. Shaken, I wondered what else my alter ego had done lately without my knowledge.

Actually, I wondered what else I had done over the past five years, since my twins were born. For it was after their arrival—just before my 35th birthday—that my mental functioning had begun its decline from pretty decent to downright unreliable, prompting me to joke, somewhat uneasily, that I must have hit "muddle age."

During that first nightmarish year of caring for twin infants, I could explain away my memory lapses and foggy thinking as the direct result of severe sleep deprivation. But, as time has passed, I continue losing sunglasses and store receipts. I still leave my purse in the house when I get into the car, and my purse in the car when I go into the house. I turn left off my street toward my boys' school when it's time to turn right and pick up my daughter at hers. I write "Pay Property Taxes" on the calendar in red ink and then rack up hundreds of dollars in late penalties. I write reminders on Post-Its and make meticulous lists of things to do, items to buy, places to go—and then arrive at my first destination only to realize that I've left my lists at home.

Then there's the morning routine, in which I help my twin boys brush their teeth and then spray an allergy medication in their noses. More mornings than I care to count, as each boy leaves the bathroom, I say, "Did I just give you your nose spray?" For I am standing there with the spray canister in one hand and the cap in the other, and for the life of me I can't remember whether I'm about to spray or just finished spraying.

One day a fellow mom of twins—plus two older singletons, bless her—stopped by to drop off an important item she'd forgotten to give me earlier. (Of course, in recounting this, I can't recall what the item was. And I'll bet she couldn't either.) She apologized, tapping her head. "I used to be sharp," she said sadly. For a few minutes we lamented the state of our mental faculties and speculated on the reasons for their decline. We cast blame squarely on the kids. With their endless chatter, petty arguments, nonstop snacking, mysterious medical maladies, and nightly homework battles—not to mention the daily challenge of locating their misplaced shoes, books, and toys—it's a minor miracle that we get them out the door each morning, and a major one that we tuck them safely into bed each night. With "just" one or even two children, it all somehow seemed more manageable, but the arrival of twins elevated multitasking to a whole new level that remains the same even as the tasks themselves change. Watching my comrade walk back to her bouncing minivan, I felt a tiny bit relieved. At least I wasn't alone.

Still, I wondered whether it's really just the kids. For years, a forty-something friend has complained about her declining memory and intellect, and she has no children. If kids aren't the culprit, maybe there's hope for regaining my cognitive abilities before my twins leave for college. One night after I'd drained the double baths, doled out double goodnight kisses, and folded double loads of laundry, I searched the Internet for other possible explanations for my muddled state of mind. I was surprised to read that hormone levels can play a critical role in women's mental acuity, and that these levels start to decline even before menopause.

This got me wondering about my own hormones, since lately I'd suffered irregular periods and debilitating monthly headaches. I made an appointment with my gynecologist, who indeed diagnosed peri-menopause—the precursor to menopause. "But I'm only thirty-nine!" I wailed. That was a little early, but not unheard of, she explained, and without treatment I could expect to suffer a whole constellation of unpleasant symptoms until true menopause begins. Then she handed me a prescription for birth control pills to tame my renegade hormones.

After a few months on the pill, some of the annoying physical symptoms had abated; even my mind seemed a little clearer. Unfortunately, though, despite trials of several brands, the headaches grew worse, and ultimately I had to give up the pill completely. Surprisingly, even that year's worth seems to have resolved the physical symptoms, at least for the time being. The cognitive troubles are another matter, however. Why, just the other day I deleted an e-mail because I didn't recognize the name of the sender, who, it turns out, is a business acquaintance with whom I'd exchanged several e-mails in the past.

I resolved to find another solution. Back at the computer, I unearthed an interesting article. A team of Yale researchers has found that stress activates protein kinase C (PKC), an enzyme that impairs short-term memory and other functions in the brain's prefrontal cortex. Because this enzyme is also active in bipolar disorder and schizophrenia, says the article, new drugs may soon be developed to inhibit PKC production.

This intrigued me. I wondered whether such a drug could someday spell relief for us multitasking moms of multiples as well. Sure, we'd still have to endure the myriad stressors—emotional, physical, and financial—of raising multiples. But, because carving out time to indulge in traditional stress-busters like bubble baths and yoga often leads to more stress, perhaps a little anti-PKC pill would be just what the doctor ordered.

One evening, Mark and I took the kids to Nina's school's open house. We drove two cars and parked on a side street so Mark could make a quick getaway with the twins when they got bored. Sure enough, I was deep in conversation with my daughter's teacher when the boys developed a giggling fit and Mark decided to leave. I waved goodbye; Nina and I would follow in the other car later.

Five minutes later, Mark burst into the classroom, breathless, boys in tow. "Someone stole both the cars!" he yelled. I paused; I knew this wasn't the best neighborhood in town, but it wasn't exactly gang turf either. I bid the perplexed teacher a hasty goodbye and followed Mark to the front of the school, where he was guiding me toward a side street. Only I could swear that we'd parked one block farther north. I ran ahead and looked. Sure enough, our cars were on the next street over, hand wipes and child safety seats intact.

I didn't know whether to laugh or cry at this turn of events. How will our multiply blessed family function with not one, but two, muddle-aged parents at its helm? I guess we'll get by somehow, if always a day or two late and a dollar or two short. But it seems we both could use that anti-PKC pill . . . or a little more estrogen.

Points to Ponder

....

Do you think your memory is less sharp since you've become a parent? Cite some examples of things you've forgotten (that you remember!).

What other symptoms of "muddle age" are you experiencing?

Do you think kids help keep us young—or age us more quickly? Why do you feel this way?

Intriguing Twins
DIETRICH AND SABINE BONHOEFFER

In 1906, Dietrich and Sabine Bonhoeffer, boy/girl twins, were born into a prominent doctor's family in a suburb of Berlin, Germany. When their older brother Walter was killed in World War I at the age of eighteen, Dietrich developed a lifelong hate for killing and war. Dietrich's strict parents expected him to be a successful doctor or lawyer, so you can imagine their reaction when he announced that he wanted to be a minister! Dietrich's parents weren't very interested in religion, but Dietrich had been reading the Bible and knew that he must pursue a different path. At the age of twenty-one, he earned a doctorate in theology *summa cum laude* and was ordained a Lutheran minister. He also began a very successful writing career. In 1930, he was invited to spend a year at Union Seminary near Harlem, New York. Hitler was beginning his rise to power when Dietrich boarded the ship.

In New York, Dietrich attended Abyssinian Baptist Church and encountered dark-skinned people for the very first time. He was fascinated by the open way in which they worshiped God and even bought recordings of gospel songs to bring back to Germany. Because of this experience, Dietrich became very intolerant of racial prejudice.

Meanwhile, in Germany, Hitler gained more and more power, and was named chancellor on January 30, 1933. Now back in his homeland, Dietrich was on the radio two days later saying, "A man who lets himself be worshiped mocks God." He was cut off by a song, and the Nazis took control of the media. Surprisingly, even the German churches supported Hitler. They hung banners bearing the swastika and started services with "Heil Hitler!" When Dietrich urged pastors to speak out against Hitler's policies, he was mostly ignored.

Soon, the troubles in Germany became personal. Dietrich's twin sister Sabine married a Jew, Gerhardt Liebholz. When Gerhardt asked Dietrich to speak at his father's funeral, Dietrich bowed to pressure and refused the request. Even though Sabine and Gerhardt later forgave him and were able to escape Germany thanks to Dietrich's assistance, it was a decision that would haunt Dietrich forever. For two years, Dietrich ran a clandestine seminary for the small number of German pastors who were against Hitler. When his actions were discovered, the students were forced into the army and Dietrich was forbidden to preach, teach, or write. Dietrich accepted an invitation to return to Union Seminary in New York, but once he was there he felt his conscience calling him back to Germany. Even though his American friends warned him against it, three weeks later Dietrich sailed on the last ship that would go to Germany before the war began.

Learning that millions of people were scheduled to be sent to death camps, a group was formed to plan Hitler's assassination. Dietrich was recruited to find support among the Allies, even though he hated the thought of killing. All attempts against Hitler's life were unsuccessful.

In 1943, Dietrich was thrown into Berlin's Tegel prison, where he was kept in solitary confinement for almost two years. Sympathetic guards brought him paper and pens and smuggled out his writings. They were later published as a book, *Letters and Papers from Prison*. Dietrich eventually ended up in a concentration camp at Buchenwald, where he brought comfort to many prisoners. When Hitler realized he was losing the war, he drew up a list of prisoners that he wanted killed before the Allies came. Dietrich was on that list. He was sent to the camp at Flossenburg, where he was put on trial and sentenced to death by hanging. Dietrich Bonhoeffer was killed on April 9, 1945, at the age of thirty-nine.

"What If I Love One Twin More Than the Other?"

Parents are often devastated to find that one child just seems more lovable to them than the other. They may see one twin as "the difficult one" and the other as more easygoing. This is not uncommon, even among singleton siblings.

Sometimes children go through phases and don't necessarily have the same temperament throughout their childhoods. One child may behave monstrously at age four, but turn into a much more lovable character by the age of six. That's why it's important not to label our kids and assume they're destined to have the same personality forever. One twin may be your (unspoken) "favorite" right now, but it could be a different story in the teen years.

As a parent, try not to be too hard on yourself when you don't always find yourself liking a child. Often, parents' feelings of frustration in these situations are directed more at themselves because they don't like how they respond to the difficult child. They may hate themselves for losing their tempers or not being as patient with this child as with the other. This makes it difficult to accept this twin as he or she is and to appreciate the good qualities.

So, how can you cope? Think of the difficult twin as a gift who will help you become a better, more patient parent. He or she is a challenge who can actually help you grow as a person and learn to cultivate your own good qualities, such as forgiveness and patience.

Also, remind yourself that there's a difference between not loving a person and not loving his or her behavior. You may not like how your "difficult" twin acts sometimes, but if you search your heart, you may find that you do, indeed, love this little person—in spite of his or her frustrating actions.

Sometimes twins act up because they need more personal attention. Try to spend more time alone with the difficult child so he or she isn't competing for your attention with the other twin. Get to know this child as an individual and find out about his interests. Seek out something special about this child that you can admire. When your child is sassy, you might tell yourself, "I was a shy kid, so I really admire how well my child knows his own needs and isn't afraid to express his opinions." Think about how these "difficult" traits might actually be a benefit later in life. The child who is very assertive or has lots of energy may actually find these qualities to be an asset as an adult.

Oftentimes, we may relate better to the child who is more like us. One child may remind you of yourself at her age, while another reminds you of your difficult father-in-law. When you're doing things together, you may naturally gravitate toward the child whose interests and temperament are more closely aligned with your own. On the other hand, you might find yourself being less tolerant of this same child's misbehavior because you notice those personality traits in your child that you dislike in yourself. Nobody likes to have a little mirror walking around, reminding them of their own personality flaws! It's important to remember that your children didn't pick their genes and personality, and they shouldn't be punished for them. Again, look for the qualities you do admire and can relate to in both children.

If you still find it tough to have equal affection for both children, it might be helpful to read some parenting books geared toward helping you raise a difficult child. They may have some great tips for helping you to better understand why your child behaves the way he or she does. With understanding come acceptance and love.

Finally, be sure to let both twins know that you admire and love them as individuals. It's never right to openly express your favoritism, even though it is natural to feel that way inside. Both children are a blessing in that they have a lot to teach you about parenting, life, and other people.

Points to Ponder

Are your twins alike or different in personality and temperament? In what ways?

Is one twin more a match to you in terms of personality or temperament? How does this affect your behavior toward this child? What do you admire most in the child who is least like you?

Have you ever felt guilty about feeling closer to one twin than the other? In what ways have you tried to bond more with the twin who's more difficult?

Have your twins acquired any labels, such as the "athletic one" or the "shy one"? How do they feel about this?

If one child is more difficult than the other, what have you learned about yourself in dealing with this child?

Twin Competition Can Get Rough!

As you've undoubtedly figured out by now, it's a common misconception that twins are so "in tune" that they always get along. In fact, the opposite is often true. Because twins, being the same age, tend to spend even more time in each other's company than other siblings, and because they are usually thrust into the same situations (same grade in school, same parties to attend, etc.), the competition between them can be even more

fierce than with non-twin siblings. As one twin described it, "We're fighting for a position of dominance!" At times they may resent that two of
them fill the place in the family where one would normally be. It's tough
to share that spotlight. It's not uncommon for any twin, at some point in
life, to glamorize how wonderful things would be without someone constantly by his or her side. Although this usually passes and twins grow to
appreciate having each other, it can lead to a lot of rivalry in the interim.
One twin who happened to be born first used to tell her sister that she (the
first twin) was the "real" child, while her twin was just her "copy." You can
imagine that comment didn't go over well with the second-born twin!

Twins mom Nancy Molter told me, "Only athletes competing for
gold medals and fame know the same level of competition that my
children show! 'Mommy, are my teeth cleaner than his?' 'Mommy, are
my training wheels a little better than hers?' 'Mommy, do you like my
painting better?' This all starts the minute they wake up in the morning with, 'Daddy, pick me up first!' At night, we close out the day
with, 'Mommy, kiss me good-night first!' It's crazy!"

Needless to say, it's important for parents to be sensitive to twins'
tendency toward competition and to allow each to be "top dog" once in
a while. Twins mom Leslie Kelley-Genson says that her friends recommend implementing "decision days." Here's how it works: "On alternate days, each twin gets a chance to call the shots, whether it's what
they have for lunch, what they watch on TV, or whether they go to the
playground or the pool. Just give each of them a day that's all theirs so
they can relax and not have to feel competitive with their twin."

It's also good to recognize your twins' uniqueness by referring to
them by their names, rather than as "the twins" or "the girls/boys."
The more twins are treated as individuals and less like a unit, the less
likely they are to engage in competition. And they may even find that
good, healthy competition can be enjoyable once in a while, as the
twins in the following story by mom Mary Brauer found.

Twins Tale

A UNIQUE COMPETITION
Mary Brauer

One afternoon, my husband and I overheard our seven-year-old twins chatting animatedly about last year's bout with the flu. "Yeah, that was great! First Dad got sick, then he passed it to me, and I threw up twenty-one times!" The other twin responded, "Uh-huh, then you gave it to me, and I threw up twenty-eight times, plus I got it all over Mom's back on the last one. That was awesome, wasn't it?"

We shuddered at the memory, and my husband responded, "Was it really that many times?" They thought for a moment and one answered, "Oh yeah, it was actually thirty-four times." Without missing a beat, the other piped up and stated, "It was forty times for me."

Twins have a unique set of circumstances that fosters competition between them. The truth of the matter is that twins begin competing the nanosecond they're conceived. For fraternal twins, it begins with who was conceived first (they can actually be conceived up to a week apart). Once they begin developing, there's jockeying for position in the womb and who can place the most strategic kicks to Mom's bladder and ribs.

Then there's intense pressure on who is designated by the medical community to be "Twin A" and "Twin B." (Twin A is usually born first, hence the reason she gets the first letter in the alphabet.)

Once they're out in the world, all of their first milestones are naturally compared because they're the same age and in the same household. It's usually known (and recorded) who smiles, rolls over, sits up, crawls, walks, and runs first.

They have an intuitive sense of how long they receive attention from their caregiver and let out heart-tugging wails if one feels left out. It seems that parents of twins are always juggling either one or two infants at a time, desperately trying to pay equal attention to both. The sad reality is that parents of twins usually harbor some hidden guilt for giving more attention to one than the other at some junction. I've rationalized it and realized that it won't do any good to feel guilty now. I'll feel guilty when it's uncovered in therapy in another twenty years.

Losing the first tooth is a milestone that fosters competition. It's not unheard of that while one twin eagerly awaits the arrival of the tooth fairy, the other twin is most likely trying to loosen up a tooth to share in the booty.

During the long potty training period, I solicited advice from other parents who cruised successfully into the dry underwear stage. I tried every suggestion possible, except for using a chart. We couldn't put a star on a chart for when each was successful on the potty because one of them went more frequently than the other.

As the school years approach, parents and educators make decisions on when to separate twins. Each set of twins is unique, but often they reach a point when it's best for them to be in separate classes. I've actually learned more about the happenings at school because my twin sons constantly compare what each did in class. Whenever I ask one of them what he did, I get the blank look and standard response, "I don't know."

As much as twins compete with each other, they also know when to turn it into an advantage. Last night we played a few games of cards. At first they fiercely competed against each other, and I won most of the hands. Once they realized this, they turned the tables on me. Suddenly, they were comparing their hands and strategizing how to beat me. And they did trounce me . . . thoroughly. As I charged them with blatant cheating and ganging up on their poor, helpless mother, I smiled inside knowing that they can effectively harness their competitive edge.

Points to Ponder

Do you think twins are more or less competitive with each other than singleton siblings? Why or why not?

In what ways do your multiples compete with each other? Is competition always unhealthy, or can it be beneficial?

What methods have you used to help your twins not be overly competitive?

Twins Trivia
IS THERE ALWAYS A "GOOD TWIN" AND A "BAD TWIN"?

Of course not! Like any two siblings, your twins are going to have differences in personality or go through different developmental stages. One may go through a stage where he's as sweet as molasses, while the other one makes you want to tear your hair out! But beware, just as you've slapped the "good" or "bad" labels on your twins, they're likely to go through a new stage in which they'll swap roles. All children have challenging periods of development. Unfortunately (or is it fortunately?), twins usually pick different times to do so.

Intriguing Twins

Lillian Gertrud Asplund

In the early morning hours of April 15, 1912, the *Titanic*—once described as "unsinkable"—went down in the North Atlantic after striking an iceberg. Fifteen hundred people died, but Lillian Gertrud Asplund, aged five, survived, along with her mother Selma and brother Felix, age three. Sadly, Lillian's fraternal twin brother, as well as her father and two other brothers, perished in the tragedy. Lillian was the last American survivor of the *Titanic* tragedy when she died at the age of ninety-nine in May 2006.

Although Lillian remembered many details of the sinking, she rarely talked about it and shied away from publicity. Her mother Selma talked about the ordeal, though, in an interview with the *Worcester Telegram & Gazette* not long after the accident. She recalled going to the upper deck after the crash and seeing icebergs all around the ship. Her husband told her and Lillian to board one of the lifeboats and smiled as he told her that he and the others would catch another one. That was the last they saw of him and the other children, except little Felix.

Lillian never married. She worked as a secretary and cared for her mother, who remained deeply troubled by the tragedy and her great loss. Selma died at the age of ninety-one in 1964—on the 52nd anniversary of the sinking.

No Longer Toddlers but Still a Challenge in Public!

Remember when your twins were toddlers and you looked forward to them getting a little older because it would be easier to control them? Think again! It doesn't matter whether they're two or ten; they're still going to make your outings a challenge—especially when you try to take them places where a little formality is called for. Going to church, attending a wedding, sitting through an awards ceremony—all are fertile ground for your little sweetie pies to be their most exasperating in public. There's no easy answer for getting them to behave. Just try to limit the non-kid-friendly activities and bring quiet things to amuse your kids, such as some new books. And make sure they've used the potty before you go! Twins mom Lynne Sella found this out the hard way when she subjected her little darlings to a prestigious event. And Holly Engel-Smothers discovered that even the video store can become a disaster zone when three kids are in tow.

Twins Tale

MESSIAH MADNESS
Lynne Sella

Every Christmas our community puts on a performance of *The Messiah*. One year, after a long absence, my parents decided to once again sing in the presentation. Not having attended since the birth of our twin daughters, my husband and I decided to go and let our daughters hear their grandparents sing.

All decked out in our best and ready for an evening of culture and refinement, we arrived early to secure good seats. With thirty minutes remaining until the beginning of the performance, my husband and I had our hands full keeping two seven-year-olds occupied. Fortunately, the singing started just before our patience ended.

The chorus began, and we all settled back in our seats. Only five minutes into it, however, one of my daughters turned to me with a strange look on her face. "Mom, I have to go to the bathroom."

"You'll have to wait," I whispered.

"But, Mom, I really have to go." The girls had attended vacation bible school in the very building in which we were sitting, so my daughter knew where the nearest bathroom could be found.

"Okay," I said, "but go very quietly." She did and soon returned.

Thoroughly enjoying the performance, I glanced over at my other daughter and was horrified to find her picking her nose. Not delicately or discreetly, but really going after it!

"Stop picking your nose!" I hissed.

"But it itches," she answered, removing her finger. She then proceeded to make the strangest faces, trying to move her nose without touching it. Rolling my eyes, I looked at my husband, hoping for some kind of reassurance that we had not made a mistake in bringing the girls to such a grownup event.

Now, my husband is an active man who rarely sits still unless there is a killer football game on television, but there he was, sitting most erect, with little beads of sweat covering his face. He looked like a caged animal waiting for the first opportunity to make good his escape. I knew at that moment I was on my own.

Forty-five minutes later, my daughter leaned over and said, "Mom, I have to go again."

"But you just went," I reminded her, hoping no one else could hear our conversation.

"I know, but I have to go again." God help me! I nodded at her and she once more walked down the aisle toward the restroom. I was thankful that she was short and did not seem to attract too much attention as she passed back and forth. After a longer stay, she returned to her seat. Within moments, I realized something was wrong.

"I got a fart coming up," she told me, panic in her eyes.

"Hold it!" I said, giving her a stern look.

"I can't," she replied, and I knew it was too late. Soon the people seated around us were being subjected to this social faux pas. It was so eye watering that they probably thought it came from my husband, rather than this adorable child. I just prayed no one thought it was mine!

Having endured the first hour of the performance, the members of my family were ready to go. I explained that it wouldn't be long until the final Hallelujah Chorus would be sung, but I didn't have the heart to tell them that it's a ten-minute song.

When the last notes were sung and the applause died down, my tribe was on its feet and out the door. I'm just grateful that no little old ladies were run over in the process. What pleasures the fine arts can bring!

Twins Tale

THE PUBLIC PUKE
Holly Engel-Smothers

The "public puke" is the true test of motherhood. It is difficult to fake a smile and the glow of motherhood when the chunks are flying. We were in Blockbuster Video, standing in line to pay for videos the other day. One of my daughters, Bailee, complained that her tummy hurt.

"We'll be home in five minutes. Hang in there. Maybe you're just hungry," I said.

"But it really hurts, Mama," whined my daughter.

As I dug out my billfold, I heard it: the undeniable sound of a child throwing up. The next few minutes seemed to happen in slow motion, but my mind was spinning. *Should I catch it before it hits the ground? Should I use my purse as a barf bag? Is anyone watching? Maybe I can just sneak out the emergency exit.*

Then I saw it: the Blockbuster Popcorn Bucket—perfect! I grabbed it and held it up to Bailee's little face. I caught most of it. Out of the corner of my eyes I saw the clerk's horrified expression. The other people in line covered their mouths. One little boy yelled, "Ewww! She's barfing, Mom!" A couple just coming in the door turned around and left with their hands over their mouths and eyes bulging. My other two kids began to wail. I saw my life flash before my eyes. And then it was all over. A deafening silence enveloped the store.

The aftermath became a complicated dance. My mind was spinning. *Do I pay for the Bucket o' Barf? Offer to clean up the floor? Still get the videos? Apologize? Or thank God for the one time I don't have to clean it up? What do I wipe Bailee's mouth with—the receipt? Can duct tape (my solution to everything) fix this mess?* Everyone was staring at me and couldn't turn away. They must have been suffering from "train wreck syndrome." They simply had to see how the gory mess turned out.

I noticed the lady behind us stepping back. She had splatters on her tennis shoes. *Oh, please,* I prayed in my mind, *let her shoes be the same ten-dollar kind I buy at Wal-Mart! Do I have to buy her new shoes? Should I just ignore the obvious splatters of today's peanut butter and jelly on her shoes?*

As if we all awoke from a spell at the same time, everyone scurried to stabilize the situation. It was like watching FEMA in action. One clerk came at me with a trash bag for the Bucket o' Barf. Another came from seemingly nowhere with spray and paper towels. The third clerk rang up the videos, reached into my purse, grabbed a five-dollar bill, and had my videos waiting for me by the door in seconds. The manager was behind me passing out free video coupons to the victims of the disaster. Someone took me by the shoulder and guided me and my kids out the door. Did the video clerks receive training in this?

Bailee had a paper towel over her mouth, and all three kids were crying. When we got in the van, I asked, "Why the tears?" Rilee answered, "Bailee threw up!" She began to cry even harder. I began to cry, too. It was only three o'clock, and my husband wouldn't be home for another three hours. *Well,* I thought to myself, *at least I've got videos to pass the time!*

Points to Ponder

What is the most embarrassing thing one or both of your twins has or have done in public?

How do you handle it when your children misbehave in public?

Have you given up any activities, such as going to church or the theater, because it's just too much trouble to bring your kids? When do you think you'll be able to resume these activities?

Tiptoeing toward Separation

When twins enter the school years, the issue of separation becomes particularly important. This is a time when twins are beginning to spread their wings and strive for independence from each other, and yet at other times they will want to be together as much as they always have. There's security in having your twin by your side. Many parents worry that their twins spend too much time together; others are alarmed when twins suddenly want their own space. Twins may request separate bedrooms at this stage, but the next day refuse to go somewhere if their twin is not invited. Twin relationships are all different, so there's no one-size-fits-all advice as to whether they should be encouraged to spend more time together or apart. While singleton children also have to learn to separate from their parents, twins have the added task of learning to separate from each other, too. So, what's a parent to do? Take a cue from the kids. Let them explore their own ways of relating—coming together and growing apart. Try not to force them to engage in the same activities or, alternately, spend unwanted time apart. Eventually, they will work out the extent of their separateness on their own, as Lisa Crystal's twin sons did.

Twins Tale

THE KEY TO CLOSENESS: TIME APART
Lisa Crystal

While pregnant with my twin boys, I was mesmerized by the intimate images of multiples that graced the pages of books and magazines: chubby infants sucking each other's fingers and toes, toothy toddlers hugging without reserve, and adorable preschoolers sharing ice cream cones. Huge, hormonal, and couch bound, I derived much-needed encouragement from those photos. As an introvert whose one child so far, a girl, was on the solitary side like me, I couldn't wait to witness the growth of this unique twin bond in my boys.

As a bonus, I figured that twins' apparent affinity for togetherness could offset some of our "start-up" costs. After reading that multiples often sleep better when bunked together in their first few months—and that even preemies are more likely to thrive in specially designed twin isolettes—I purchased one crib for the time being. I couldn't wait to take photos of my babies snuggled in their nest for two.

The first hint that my own twins might be less than picture perfect came in my hospital bed, shortly after their births. Maneuvering around my intravenous tubes, I cuddled each baby individually, and then, with a pillow protecting my C-section incision, my husband arranged Ian and Graham in my lap so we three could snuggle.

Oh, the squeaks of protest! They squirmed in unison, four tiny fists flailing. Entranced, I realized that I had felt these precise movements within me over the past months. Clearly they weren't happy now. Perhaps they were sick of each other's company after sharing such close quarters all those months. I rested Ian in my lap and lifted Graham to my shoulder, where he immediately relaxed and nestled comfortably. I looked down at Ian and he gazed back at me—sternly, it seemed. And it occurred to me that my twins didn't want each other. They wanted me, and they wanted their own turf.

My suspicions were quickly borne out at home. Whether arranged feet to feet, head to head, head to feet, or side by side, my sons protested their single lair. I tried settling one in the crib, and then sneaking in the other. When the first sensed the intruder, he became indignant, matching his brother grunt for outraged grunt. They kicked and punched, squirmed and fumed, dashing my fantasies of blissful coexistence.

By the time they were six months old, Graham and Ian had never slept together in a crib, sucked each other's fingers, or shown the slightest predilection for any other form of togetherness. Placed too close on the floor, one would clutch at the other's wisps of hair while that one yelped in protest. Simultaneous nursing could be tolerated only in the football hold, with heads positioned as far apart as possible—no crisscrossing or touching of body parts allowed. Even then, it was a competitive exercise involving much gasping and slurping. It seemed that each baby was determined to out-suck his brother.

By seven months, it was clear my sons needed something I had figured wouldn't be on the radar for at least a decade: their own rooms. Two cribs simply did not fit in their single small room, and our efforts to get them to sleep for longer stretches at night were stymied by their growing ability to rouse each other with their enhanced lung capacities. We moved into a larger house and transformed the intended study into temporary quarters for one of the boys.

Once the boys were ensconced in separate rooms, nights became more peaceful. And the unexpected happened: they became buddies. Perched in their highchairs, each baby would watch the other intently while sampling a new food, awaiting his brother's reaction before deciding his own. Seated on the floor, they'd roll their clicking toy school buses back and forth in unison. When they learned how to scoot on their bottoms—their version of crawling—they followed each other from room to room, taking special delight in sharing a giggle in one boy's bedroom before scooting back down the hall to the other's.

At nineteen months, after much parental fretting over the boys' failure to take a single step, Graham—the twin who had faced more physical challenges and delays in reaching milestones—finally pulled himself up and tottered across the room. Ian took one look and within fifteen seconds was careening over to join him—leading me to wonder whether he had actually been able to walk for some time. Perhaps he'd forsaken mobility in favor of something he deemed more important: solidarity with his brother.

In the years since, a relationship that at first seemed destined to be one of grudging tolerance has evolved into a fiercely loyal bond. In a simple card game, my boys play and play, and play again, until their scores are even—the goal being not to triumph over each other, but to rejoice in their dual accomplishments. They embrace anxiously before separating to run errands with a parent, spend the shopping trip searching for something special to bring back to the other—and greet each other like long-lost lovers being reunited after their hour apart. At seven years, they still unabashedly reach for each other's hand when out on a walk, synchronizing their steps and expounding on subjects often meaningful only to them. They confer and plot and discuss and analyze as they perform flips off the couch or lie on the floor or swing in the backyard hammock. They collaborate in comfortable silence on their rudimentary songwriting—deciding by unspoken agreement who will type the lyrics, who will scratch beats on the DJ mixer, and who will man the microphone.

And in the midst of all this, people sometimes ask why Graham and Ian still have separate rooms. Given their compatibility, wouldn't it make sense to finally move the "study" out of the corner of the master bedroom?

In truth, it's been tempting: I've often wondered whether I'd sleep better without reams of paper and a humming hard drive stationed three feet from my bed. But I've come to believe that my boys' separate rooms are fundamental to both their sense of self and their sense of twinship. They take pride in their own space: Each boy's room is painted a color of his own choosing, features his favorite posters, and is stocked with the books he alone selected at the library or bookstore. Each boy must ask before entering his brother's room or borrowing one of the objects that reside there. Most importantly, even at the advanced age of seven—long past the traditional napping stage—every afternoon each boy retires to his own room for about an hour to read, doodle, or just contemplate the ceiling, free of the opinions and exhortations of his brother. They then emerge from their respective spaces calm, refreshed, and ready for several more hours of intense togetherness largely devoid of antipathy. This respite has become so essential to their well-being that they actually ask for a "nap" if one isn't offered. And, on the days when there simply is no time, friendly banter can turn to petty arguing, and heartfelt sharing give way to unceremonious grabbing.

This all makes sense to me. After all, who among us can cheerfully endure the constant companionship of another, even under the most favorable circumstances? We all need a break from even our nearest and dearest to reflect and muse, to stew and worry, and to fantasize and dream free of the duty to interact. Until kindergarten, twins' daytime naps offer that essential downtime; when they're teens, twins may seek their own refuge in an MP3 player or a novel. It is those who fall in the middle—essentially grade-school age—who need encouragement and opportunity to separate, particularly if they also share a classroom.

Recently I found myself explaining this theory to an acquaintance who was lamenting her own six-year-old twins' behavior, which seemed to deteriorate over the course of the day. A separate rest time wasn't possible, she said, because her twins share a room. I suggested that one twin claim a corner of the living room or the home office for an hour; they could even alternate days in which one used the bedroom and one the other location. A week later she reported back with good news: That daily separation had quickly become a godsend to her twins, and to everyone in the family.

And so now I type this on a computer that will probably reside next to my underwear drawer until my daughter leaves for college and frees up another room. But I don't mind. Pinned above the desk is a photo of my boys peering playfully from under the blanket of one of their beds, where they like to cuddle on weekend mornings before beginning another day marked by tender moments both together and apart.

Points to Ponder

Would you say that your twins are closer to each other than other siblings, or do you see no difference between their relationship and other sibling relationships?

What signs have your twins shown of desiring more separateness, like requesting their own rooms or wanting to spend time alone?

Do you ever worry that your twins spend too much time together or, alternately, that they're not as close as you thought they'd be?

Twins Trivia

ARE CONJOINED TWINS MORE LIKELY AMONG CERTAIN ETHNIC GROUPS?

Conjoined twins (also known as Siamese twins) are a form of monozygotic (identical) twins. They occur at the same rate throughout the world. No one really knows why an egg splits (whether completely or not, as in the case of conjoined twins), and this phenomenon doesn't seem to be affected by maternal age, ethnicity, heredity, hormonal treatments, or any other factors that can result in fraternal twins. For some reason, though, conjoined twins are more likely to be female, but again, the reasons are unknown. Are more female conjoined twins actually conceived, or is it just that more of them actually survive? Scientists are still examining this issue.

Intriguing Twins
BILLY AND BENNY MCCRARY

It's not uncommon to hear about twins being small in size. They're frequently born prematurely and take a while to catch up to other kids. It's much more unusual, therefore, to hear about "big" twins—those whose size far surpasses that of other children. That's why the story of twins Billy and Benny McCrary is so fascinating. You see, these boys were hospitalized at a young age with German measles, and their illness left an unusual side effect: They couldn't stop gaining weight! Doctors believe the measles resulted in damage to their pituitary glands, causing them to weigh more than two hundred pounds each by the age of ten. At sixteen, they both weighed more than six hundred pounds apiece. But that didn't stop these amazing twins from leading exciting and interesting lives!

Their parents bought a farm, hoping the twins would burn off some calories through hard labor, but it didn't work. Billy and Benny dropped out of high school in Hendersonville, North Carolina, to work as cattle branders in Texas. They became famous when photographer John Page took a picture of the plus-size twins riding minibikes. This well-known photo landed them in *Life* magazine, as well as in the *Guinness Book of World Records* as the world's largest twins (weighing more than eight hundred pounds each at the time). This instant fame would take them a long way!

The Honda Motorcycle Company hired the twins to drive a promotional tour on their minibikes from New York to Los Angeles. They drove one hundred miles each day for thirty days, stopping at Holiday Inns each night and signing autographs at Honda dealerships. Along the way, they attended a wrestling match in El Paso, Texas, where a man named Gory Guerrero offered to train them as wrestlers. After they completed their training, their careers took off and they hit the road.

While the twins were wrestling in Japan, the announcers had a hard time pronouncing McCreary, so they changed their last name to the more common McGuire. Billy and Benny traveled around the world wrestling and even appeared on *The Tonight Show* several times. They had a show in Las Vegas, where they would tell jokes with four-hundred-pound dancers and play their trumpets.

Tragically, Billy died in 1979 after sustaining injuries while performing a daredevil stunt on his minibike at Niagara Falls. Benny had the world's largest granite gravestone placed on Billy's grave in Hendersonville, North Carolina. It's thirteen feet wide and weighs three tons. Benny continued to wrestle for a time after Billy's death and then bought a pawnshop and became an auctioneer. In 1998 he and his wife Tammie took jobs with the Christian Golfers Ministry. Benny died at age fifty-four of heart failure.

Engraved on the famous twins' giant tombstones are pictures of their beloved minibikes and words proclaiming them the world's largest twins. Billy and Benny were truly "larger than life" twins. But then, as parents of multiples know, all twins are special!

School's Out . . . It's Vacation Time!

What parent hasn't heard the wailing from the back seat, "Are we there yet?" or "I have to go to the bathroom" (for the third time in an hour)? It's enough for any parents to wish they'd dropped the kids off at Grandma's and headed for a quiet, parents-only cruise! But family vacations are the stuff of which wonderful memories are made. The best way to enjoy them is to lower your expectations. Don't expect everything to go smoothly. Don't expect all of your plans to go perfectly. In fact, don't expect anything at all! Just go with the flow. You're away from work and the drudgeries of home. Enjoy yourself and ignore the whining.

Good preparation is the key to a successful trip. Take the worries out of packing by getting the kids to help out! Nancy Johnson, mom of triplets, has had great success with this technique: "I give each child a checklist of what to pack (for example, three pairs of shorts, five T-shirts, two 'nice' shirts, five pairs of socks, etc.) and a laundry basket. They load up all the items on the list and put them in the laundry basket. Then, I can load the suitcase from the basket, checking that everything is there. This gives me the help I need, but it also gives my kids a sense of independence because they can make their own choices and are helping. My triplets have been helping me pack since they were four years old!"

You'll also need to pack plenty of things to do along the way, especially if you've planned a road trip. Bring lots of new toys and games and dole them out slowly, not all on the first day. (Check your local dollar store for inexpensive options.) Ditto for snacks. And don't be a marathon driver and expect the kids to sit in the car for ten hours. Take lots of breaks. Consider splitting up the trip by visiting places along the way. Every town you pass through is a new destination to be discovered! Sometimes interesting things can be found off the beaten path rather than in a guidebook. The kids will be talking for years to come about the little fish they saw jumping in a pond or the creaky old bridge you crossed over. These unexpected pleasures often have more impact than a sighting of Mickey Mouse or a stop at a fast-food restaurant.

When you've reached a sightseeing destination, don't try to pack in as many activities as possible. Tired kids get cranky and irritable (and so do adults!). Schedule a couple of days during your trip for just relaxing at the beach or hanging around the cabin or hotel pool. Enjoy your time together! Here are a few more ideas for making your vacation fun with twins.

Twins Tips
ROAD-TRIPPING WITH MULTIPLES

- Kids get more excited about the destination when they're given a chance to help plan it. Consider giving each child the choice of a "must do" event that they can plan for the whole family. If Sara knows she'll get to see her theme park and Joey knows the baseball stadium is on the agenda, they'll be more willing to go along with the plans that you have made.

- Encourage your twins to be collectors! Buy photo albums or scrapbooks in which they can collect postcards from each place you visit. Some kids like to collect charms for a special bracelet, pins to fasten on their backpacks, "squashed pennies," or baseball caps.

- Avoid the "he always gets the best seat" argument by assigning seating and sleeping arrangements ahead of time. If both kids covet the same position, perhaps they can trade off each day. Laying down the ground rules ahead of time will help minimize the squabbling.

- Encourage your multiples to take pictures by giving each an inexpensive or throwaway camera. Teach them that the best shots don't come through the window of a moving car! Develop some of the pictures at a one-hour photo place so the kids can arrange them in their albums during the long drive.

- Pack a first-aid kit, including medicine for carsickness. (Talk to your pediatrician about children's dosages.) Nothing ruins a car trip more quickly than having to inhale the smell of vomit all the way!

- Consider buying bright, matching T-shirts for the whole family so you can easily identify each other in crowded places. Make sure to teach your twins about what to do if you get separated and arrange for a meeting place.

Points to Ponder

Have you gone on vacation with your twins yet? How did it go? What went wrong? What worked out well?

What are your future plans for vacationing with your twins? What preparations will you make to help things run smoothly?

What special memories do you have of family vacations from when you were growing up?

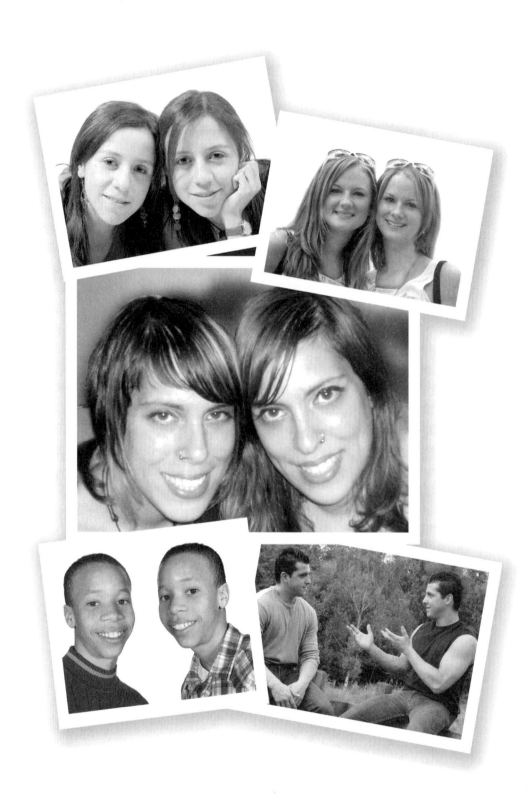

Part 4

Twin Tweens and Teens
(Ages 12–17)

If you're raising teenage twins, I have one piece of advice for you: Go back and read the toddler chapter. Really! Have you ever noticed how kids seem to revert to their toddler ways when they hit the teen years? I'm currently raising two (singleton) teenagers along with toddler twins, so I know what I'm talking about! Let's do a comparison:

	Toddlers	Teenagers
Have tantrums when they don't get their way	Yes	Yes
Are sassy and disobedient	Yes	Yes
Have a lot to learn about life!	Yes	Yes
Drive parents crazy	Yes	Yes
Are finicky eaters	Yes	Yes
Lack motivation to behave or follow instruction	Yes	Yes
Hate to go to bed at night	Yes	Yes
Grow like weeds	Yes	Yes
Fight with their siblings	Yes	Yes

See what I mean? Teenagers are just toddlers in bigger clothes. Why didn't we cherish the blissful elementary school years while we could? But alas, the teen years arrive all too quickly, so we might as well make the best of them. It's not easy, though, when you've got double hormones and double sass to deal with! And, while most teenagers normally struggle with identity issues, this becomes more complex for twins who yearn even more to be recognized for themselves and not as part of a matched set. You may find one or both of them making a sudden and unexpected dash for independence and separation from their twin . . . or finding that they appreciate having a twin even more when issues of popularity, peer pressure, and puberty assail them. It's a time of change for the twin relationship (as well as the parent–teen relationship!), so it's especially important to have some coping skills in place during the tween and teen years.

The Advantages of Being Twins in Adolescence

- Twins are never alone. When they feel that their peers have rejected them, they always have a friend at home who knows and loves them for themselves.
- Twins have more empathy for others because they've been thinking about another person's feelings ever since they were very young. This often makes twin teens more compassionate toward others.
- Twins can play off each other's strengths. If one twin is better at math and another at English, they can help each other study or learn the material.
- Twins can be each other's sounding boards. Teens often feel they have no one to talk to. Having a twin provides another set of ears from someone who understands what it's like to be a teen.
- Twins have more power as a team. When they want something, such as a new gaming system or a trip, it's much tougher for parents or grandparents to resist their twins' double pleas!

Points to Ponder

What would your twins say are some additional advantages to being a twin?

Do you think that having a twin has helped your children adjust to peer scrutiny and pressure?

Have your twins grown closer together or further apart as they've entered adolescence? Why do you think this has happened?

The Disadvantages of Being Twins in Adolescence

- During adolescence, all teens struggle to form an identity separate from their parents. Twins have the additional job of forging an identity that makes them different from their twin.

- At a time when kids don't like to be seen as "different," being a twin really makes them stand out from the crowd. Sometimes they worry that it makes them "weird."
- People often treat twins as a unit and don't appreciate them as individuals. Twins resent being called "The Smith Twins" rather than "Cara" and "Beth."
- Teenagers frequently strive for more privacy, which is difficult to find when they're a twin. Being the same age naturally means that they're both included in the same activities. If they share a room, it's even more difficult for twins to find distance from each other.
- Competition may increase. As teenagers develop greater competency in certain areas, one twin may feel like a failure if her twin excels in something that she doesn't.

Points to Ponder

What would your twins say are some additional disadvantages to being a twin?

Do your twins like or dislike being twins now that they're teenagers?

Have your twins asked for more privacy as teenagers? Do they desire separate rooms or want their twin left out of certain activities?

Talking with Moms Who Have Been There

As I write this, I currently have two teenagers in the house, ages seventeen and fourteen. Whenever I encounter problems with them, my mind naturally gasps in horror at the thought: *How will I ever manage with twins going through adolescence at the same pace?* It's tough for me to imagine two kids advancing through the same stages and levels of maturity in the teen years simultaneously. I have a feeling it won't be quite the same as raising two singleton teens. With that in mind, I went to the "experts" and talked to a couple of moms who have already navigated their way through the teen years with their twins. Pat Enriquez and Bette Ade were kind enough to answer the following questions about raising their now-grown twin girls as adolescents.

Twins Tale

AN INTERVIEW WITH TWO MOMS WHO HAVE
SURVIVED THE TEEN YEARS WITH TWINS
Susan Heim with Pat Enriquez and Bette Ade

Are your twins identical or fraternal?

Pat: Identical.

Bette: Maternally identical, but paternally fraternal. The theory is that one egg splits, and then the two eggs are fertilized by different sperm, thus explaining differences in height, etc. Our twins pass all the tests for being identical except for a three-inch height difference.

Would your twins say that being a twin was an advantage or a disadvantage in the teen years?

Pat: My girls have told me that they never felt lonely and always had someone there to talk to who would understand.

Bette: Both girls agreed that being twins was an advantage because they always had a friend, someone in whom they could confide, someone close. The disadvantage was that people did not make an effort to tell them apart. (Interestingly, we had neighbors whose three-year-old son had Down syndrome. He could tell them apart— and still can in his mid-thirties, even when their teachers at school couldn't tell the difference between them.)

Were your twins competitive as teenagers?

Pat: Not at all. They always supported each other, no matter what they were doing.

Bette: Karen says no; Karla says yes. (Go figure!) A traumatic event for me as a mother was when Karla and Karen played against each other in a basketball game their senior year in high school. Karen had married the summer before her senior year (with our permission, by the way—she and Jeff celebrated their 25th wedding anniversary last August) and attended a different school from her previous years with Karla. As seniors, they were both team captains at this tournament. Their teammates kept telling the referees that they were twins, but of course, the refs didn't believe the story. K & K got very rough with each other, poking, bumping, etc., and the refs kept saying, "Ladies, ladies!" I was expecting technical fouls against one or both of them. I don't remember who won. Karen remembers that she played her best game ever, and Karla remembers that her team "smoked" Karen's.

Did your twins become closer as teens, or did they grow apart in a quest to form their own identities?

Pat: They were always glued at the hip and still are at the age of twenty-six!

Bette: They were close as teens, but with Karen being married at seventeen and then Karla going off to university at eighteen, they naturally were not as close. But even now, at forty-two, they talk often and see each other occasionally. (They live a couple of hours apart.)

Do you feel it was tougher to raise two teenagers at once than it would have been with just one?

Pat: Yes, they always stuck together and always played good cop/bad cop with us. One would beg for something, and if we didn't give in, she would argue with us. There would be a yelling match, and she would storm out of the room. Then the other twin would come in the room and tell us that her sister was wrong for arguing with us, and she realizes we are sticking to our guns because we love them, but . . . (The begging would then continue until we gave in!)

Bette: Actually, we raised three at one time, as our oldest daughter was twenty-two months older than the twins. The girls didn't suffer too much sibling rivalry, for which we are very thankful.

In what ways was it easier to raise teenage twins than it might have been with just one?

Pat: Whenever they went out, we knew they were together, so it felt safer to us. We always felt that if one of them were going to do something dumb that the other one would hopefully stop her.

Bette: My husband and I were only children, so I was very happy that we had more than one. (I, for one, was very spoiled, etc., as an only child, so we eliminated that problem by having three children!)

Did your teen twins share a bedroom or have separate ones? How did this arrangement work out?

Pat: We bought a bigger house so they could have their own rooms. (They were six years old.) They constantly left their rooms to sleep together; they just wanted to be together. We threatened them after approximately a year of this that if they didn't sleep in their own rooms, we were going to use one room as an office. They told us to take the room because they wanted to stay together. We made our office, and they stayed together for the rest of their time living at home. They went to college, came back home for a few years, and finally, at age twenty-five, moved to Philadelphia—where they are still roommates, but now they have their own rooms.

Bette: Our twins shared a bedroom, and our singleton had a bedroom to herself. Of course, when Karen married, Karla had the bedroom to herself.

Did your teen twins have the same friends or different friends (or both)?

Pat: They had all the same friends, and their boyfriends were usually good friends with each other.

Bette: They had mutual friends, but their "best friends" were different.

Did you ever feel that your teen twins were too close for their own good?

Pat: Yes, and I still feel that way. I can't imagine them really living apart.

Bette: No, they were very independent, but close. There was never any worry about them being isolated [from others].

What complaints did your teen twins have about being twins?

Pat: They complained when people didn't know them apart. That really still bothers them. They hated when people spoke about one of them and always said "they." A lot of people feel they are the same person, and this really bugs them.

Bette: People not trying to tell them apart. Sometimes being treated as a set, rather than as individuals.

Do you have any tips for other parents raising teenage twins?

Pat: Try to make everybody know they are individuals and not the same person. As they got older, my girls tried so hard not to look alike. The worst part was that one of them grew dreadlocks (ugh!) and the other one has long, shiny hair—but people still got them confused! Thank God, she finally cut off the dreads . . .

Bette: Enjoy them. Pray for you and them. *Try* to be fair. Since I was very active in Dallas MOTC and later organized Texas Mothers of Multiples, I tried to balance things by always being "room mother" for Evelyn's (my oldest daughter's) classes.

Is there anything else you'd like to say about raising teenage twins?

Pat: Enjoy them when they are young. Hold your breath when they become teenagers, and be glad when they turn twenty-five and finally appreciate their parents!

Bette: God gives us what we can handle. I really feel that if you cannot handle what you are given, you might need to reconnect to the "Source."

Points to Ponder

What information in this interview really hit home with you and why?

Have you talked with other parents of twin teens about their experiences? What have you learned from them?

If you've raised other kids before your twin teens, how was that experience the same and different during their teen years?

Intriguing Twins
CELEBRITY TWINS

Mario Andretti	Jill Hennessy
Karen Black	Ashton Kutcher
Jose Canseco	Alanis Morissette
Aaron Carter	Tia and Tamera Mowry
Ann B. Davis	Mary-Kate and Ashley Olsen
Vin Diesel	Alexandra Paul
John Elway	Isabella Rossellini
Horace Grant	Kiefer Sutherland
Deidre Hall	Sawyer and Sullivan Sweeten
Linda Hamilton	Billy Dee Williams
Paul and Morgan Hamm	

Are Your Teens Embarrassed about Being Twins?

Every parent knows that just standing next to their teens in front of their friends at the movie theater is cause for acute embarrassment. Teens are at an age when they want to fit in and win their peers' approval, and their "uncool" parents hanging around them don't make them look good. But sometimes it's not just parents—or dopey kid brothers—who are a source of embarrassment. Having a twin can be embarrassing, too! Being a twin makes a teen *different*—and that's not always what they want. Plus, when other kids start asking them questions about being a twin, it may cause them to feel like a freak, as if there's something weird about having a twin brother or sister. There's also the "cuteness factor." Twins, especially identical twins, are often viewed by society as being "cute." Most teens definitely don't want to wear that label! And it can be exasperating when their peers just refer to them as "the Heim twins" instead of using their first names. In some cases, twins may even be mean to each other in an effort to separate and show other teens that they're not attached at the hip. Naturally, this can cause problems between them, particularly if one twin wishes to remain close and the other doesn't.

Unfortunately, this is just one of the many phases that teen twins will pass through. There's not much you can do except wait it out and not let any mean-spiritedness get out of hand. Most adolescent twins grow close again once they reach adulthood and aren't so concerned about their image in the eyes of others. Just as they'll one day decide that their parents aren't so "geeky" after all, so, too, will they realize that having a twin is a real blessing.

Points to Ponder

Do your twins get easily embarrassed by your presence? How does this make you feel?

Have your twins shown any embarrassment about being a twin?

If they're embarrassed about being a multiple, how do your twins express this? Have they begun to treat each other badly or seek more separation?

Twins Trivia

WHY ARE IDENTICAL TWINS VALUABLE TO SCIENTIFIC RESEARCH?

All of the genes in the DNA of identical twins are the same, so if a scientist wants to test whether a particular trait or disease is caused by the environment or genes, twins make ideal study subjects. Because their genes are identical, any differences between twins are most likely caused by the environment. (Fraternal twins, on the other hand, are not good study subjects because their genes are no more similar than the genes of any other brothers and sisters.)

Every year, researchers travel to Twinsburg, Ohio, for their annual Twins Days Festival. More than three thousand twins gather there every year, so scientists set up booths at the festival to recruit identical twins for their studies. Each year, twelve scientists are allowed to conduct studies in exchange for paying a few hundred dollars for a place at the festival. Researchers say this is still a bargain because if they tested twins in the general population, it would cost them more to recruit twins through advertisements, screen them, and pay any related travel expenses. The twins at the festival usually like the idea of being subjects in valuable research and often wait in line for hours for the chance to be in a scientific study.

Dealing with Teenage Twins' "Conspiracies"

Twins have a distinct advantage when they want something badly enough—they can team up on you! This can be especially effective when you've been approached alone (without your partner) and are being coerced by two very convincing charmers. Of course, sometimes this is not a conscious technique with twins. They don't necessarily think to themselves, *She can't say no with two of us ganging up on her!* But nevertheless, it's a difficult tactic to resist. And, when they truly plot and plan to overpower you, well, you'll need all your emotional strength to stand your ground!

For instance, if one twin happens to get home after curfew, he might convince his co-twin to corroborate his story that he was helping a friend with a flat tire. Or, if one twin tends to get in trouble more than the other, she may use her sister—whom you're more likely to believe—to plead her case. Another scenario is when one works on Mom and the other works on Dad to win an argument.

Is this starting to remind you of your twins' toddler years, when they combined their skills to scale the playpen walls or get into the dishwasher? Yes, two minds are definitely better than one, and twins aren't afraid to use theirs together—especially during the teen years.

You can discourage your teens from employing these techniques by reminding them to think of themselves as part of a family, rather than us (the twins) against them (the parents). And encourage your twins to explore separate pursuits and pleasures, thus reinforcing the fact that they are not one unit and must be responsible for their own actions—and the consequences of them. Finally, be firm about enforcing the household rules. For the ones that are particularly important to you—no drugs, sticking with curfew, no driving with friends, etc.—make it clear that you won't be persuaded not to punish through the arguments of one twin defending the other. Most twins want to be treated as individuals, so this is a good opportunity to stress that you plan to do just that—in every circumstance.

Do your twins tend to gang up on you when they're trying to persuade you to grant a privilege or halt a punishment?

Would you consider yourself a "softie" who frequently gives in to these conspiracies, or do you pride yourself on holding firm in the face of them?

In what ways have you discouraged your twins from engaging in conspiracies?

The Old "Switcheroo"

If your twins are identical, chances are they're going to try the old "switcheroo" at least once in their lives. Who can resist the urge to change their identity and fool someone? Of course, we must explain to our twins that it is never okay to do this when issues like tests are involved, but otherwise, it can be great fun and a real advantage for identical twins. Fraternal twins are rarely allowed this treat, as they can look quite different. This is especially difficult for boy/girl twins, of course. Now that I think of it, though, I did hear of a set of boy/girl twins who dressed up as each other for Halloween! (If your boy/girl twins try this at any other time of the year, however, you might wish to consider counseling!) Of course, sometimes pulling the old "switcheroo" can be unintentional, as twins Nicole and Janine found out in this next anecdote sent in by their mom.

Twins Tale

SWAPPING DATES
Pat Enriquez

When my twin girls, Nicole and Janine, were about fourteen years old, they went to the movies with a bunch of kids—including a brand-new boyfriend for Nicole. As they got into their seats, the boy sat next to Janine and put his arm around her. Janine was dying inside because she knew he thought she was Nicole, and she was afraid that he might try to kiss her! They didn't want to embarrass the young man, however, so the girls went into the rest room and exchanged blouses. Then Nicole sat next to her date, and he never knew the difference! By the way, he did kiss her . . .

Points to Ponder

....

Have your twins ever pulled the old "switcheroo"? If so, what were the circumstances?

Do your teenage twins get tired of people mixing them up? Do they try to counteract this in any way, such as changing their appearance?

Have your twins ever fooled *you* by intentionally switching identities?

Intriguing Twins
ELOISE AND LOUISE BOWLES

Most likely you've read the famous "Hints from Heloise" column, but did you know that it was started by an identical twin? Eloise Bowles and her sister Louise were born on May 4, 1919. Their mother Amelia also had a twin, named Ophelia!

Eloise and Louise were considered "mirror-image" twins and had a lot of fun with this trait in high school. They would play tricks on their dates and even attend each other's classes! Unfortunately, they got caught when Louise accidentally put her name on a paper that was supposed to be written by Eloise.

Although the twins were very competitive, they were also close, and their relationship inspired them to become entrepreneurs. When Eloise was living with her husband in Hawaii, where he was stationed as a captain in the Army Air Forces, she decided that the local newspaper, the *Honolulu Advertiser,* needed a column targeted to housewives. She pitched her idea to the newspaper editor and even offered to work for free for a month to see if the column would take off. They called the column "The Readers' Exchange," and it became an instant hit. It was picked up by King Features Syndicate in 1961 and renamed "Hints from Heloise." (An "H" was added to Eloise's name for its alliterative effect.)

Heloise also painted, wrote and published books and poetry, and wrote a song called "There Are No Phones to Heaven." Meanwhile, her twin Louise enjoyed her own success as an artist.

Heloise died on December 28, 1977. Most people at the funeral didn't realize she was a twin, so imagine their shock upon seeing her sister Louise at the service. The mourners thought Heloise had risen from the dead! Heloise's lawyer was also taken aback at the sight of Louise at the reading of the will.

Heloise's legacy continues, as her daughter Poncé now writes the "Hints from Heloise" column. Heloise's tombstone reads: "Heloise, Every Housewife's Friend."

Twins Trivia
WHAT ARE MIRROR-IMAGE TWINS?

Mirror-image twins are identical twins that result from the splitting of the fertilized egg late in the embryonic stage. About 25 percent of identical twins are classified as "mirror-image," and of the 6.3 billion people in the world, only 5 million are mirror-image twins. How do you know if you're looking at mirror-image twins? Well, if you have them face each other, certain traits will match up as if one were looking into a mirror. For example, their cowlicks may match (one on the left side of the head; one on the right side), or one may be left-handed and the other right-handed.

Striving for Independence

Children often strive for more independence when they enter adolescence and this can be especially true for twins. Because they're known to others as "the twins," they are often expected to think and act alike. But teen twins often resent being lumped together. They want to be seen as special because of their own unique qualities and personalities, not just because they happen to have a twin.

Twins are often seen as a "unit" in school, as well. If one twin is good in math, teachers expect the other twin to do just as well in that subject. If one is a basketball star, the other feels great pressure to excel in sports, too. Therefore, it's especially important for teen twins' self-worth that they be encouraged to develop their own interests and talents. Never insist that both twins participate in the same sports or extracurricular activities if they don't want to. If they're both invited to a particular event, make sure you consult them individually about it and allow each of them to make her own decision as to whether they'll attend. Praise them individually, not as a unit.

Most of all, don't be overly concerned if your twins suddenly make a strike for independence. Some twins grow even closer during adolescence, as they find it easier to deal with pressures with a sibling by their side, but many begin to shed the "twin" label and are ready to shine on their own. This is a natural milestone and should, in fact, be encouraged. They will soon be out in the world as adults and must function without their twin by their side.

Points to Ponder

Do your twins complain about being seen as "the twins" instead of as individuals?

What signs have your twins shown that they are striving for independence?

In what ways do you encourage your twins to develop their own individual strengths and talents?

Spending One-on-One Time with Your Twins

It's a great idea to help your teenagers feel special by spending quality time alone with each child. In this way, your twins get your undivided attention, at least for a while. Think of it this way: Would you really want your spouse to accompany you everywhere you go? Of course not! If you love browsing antique shops and your husband doesn't, you'll have a more enjoyable time without him. If you love to go to baseball games and they put your wife to sleep, wouldn't you rather go by yourself or with some buddies? It's the same with twins. Sometimes they'd just rather be without their sibling for a while so they can engage in activities that they enjoy. So, schedule "dates" with each child alone and let him or her pick the event for the day. Twins mom Mary Reeves told me, "We make an effort to plan specific 'dates' for each girl to spend one-on-one time with either Mom or Dad. This usually is a lunch date, but sometimes involves shopping for something they need or want, too. It is really nice to focus on just one and be able to have a conversation without interruption. Our last Date Day was specifically requested by one of the girls because she really needed Mom all to herself for a while." One of your daughters might want to go shopping on her date, while the other might prefer a movie. One son might want to go out for burgers, while the other is interested in a hockey game. An added benefit is that your twins are more likely to open up to you without a sibling listening in. This is a good time to talk to your twins alone about their hopes for the future, their worries and concerns, and their interests. Point out the things that you like about them individually, and let your multiples know they're special in their own ways. And enjoy these one-on-one times with them while you can. As triplets mom Pam Pace found out, they come to an end all too quickly.

Twins Tale
BRANDI'S CHOICE
Pam Pace

Well, it finally happened! I knew it would someday, just not so soon. My daughter has chosen to be with her friend over me. Pardon me while I sob . . . okay. I am going to try to hold it together while I write this article! I can't believe it. We had the "date" booked for two weeks. A trip to the hairdresser for a nice trim, and then off to our favorite Thai place, just mother and daughter. We would sip herbal tea, try some different foods, and chat forever. Just the two of us. I had been looking forward to this day for some time. Not only do I love the place she chose to eat, but I truly love being with my preteen daughter, Brandi. I love being with *all* of my daughters, but there is just something special about having one-on-one time with them. They say things they wouldn't dare say in front of their siblings or the whole family, and I can focus on just them.

My husband and I have made it a point to "date" our children since they were about two years of age. In those days, it may have only meant a trip to the grocery store with Mom, but it was time away from the chaos and noise of the house and their siblings. They would have Mom or Dad all to themselves (even it was only for thirty or forty minutes). It was precious then, and it is even more precious now. The older they get, the more they become like "little grownups" and they can discuss their feelings about life and just about anything, just like a good friend. I was really loving this age of preteen-hood—that is, until now.

We had just returned from the boys' soccer games, and as soon as we walked in the door, Bailey announced that Devon had called and wanted Brandi to sleep over Friday night. Brandi looked at me, and I looked at her. I said, "Brandi, that is our date night." She said, "I know, Mom, but I really, really want to go!" I gulped and tried to think of a way she could go and still make her hair appointment. I suggested that she go to her friend's house after school and play for a while, and then I could pick up her and her girlfriend in time for the hair appointment and return them both for the sleepover. Brandi squealed with joy as she relayed the message to her friend over the phone.

Brandi was so happy that she came over and hugged me. Then her smile turned to a sad face. "But, Mom," she said sadly, "I will miss our date. Can we do it Saturday night instead?" I said, "No, honey, Daddy and I have a date then." I told her that I was sad, too, but that I under-stood she wanted to be with her friend. I struggled to pull her up onto my lap as her feet dragged the ground. I held her tight and told her that I knew a day like today would come. As I stroked her long, beautiful blonde hair, I remarked that I knew the day would come when she would rather be with her friends than with me or her dad. I told her that it made me sad, but that I didn't want her to feel bad for me. It was just part of being a mom.

I have heard from my friends who have older children about how painful this process can be, but this mom just wasn't ready for this day to come. Not yet. It seems like just yesterday that she was in diapers and biting her sister! They grow up so fast! So, for all of you moms and dads wishing your little ones would hurry and grow up, don't wish too hard. Before you know it, they will! And, yes, you'll miss those crazy baby days when your little ones only wanted to be with you.

Points to Ponder

What interests do your twins have apart from each other?

Do you try to do things with your twins individually at times? What kinds of things have you done or would you like to do with them?

If you schedule "dates" with your kids, what benefits have you seen for them—and for you? Do you think it's a good idea to schedule time alone with each twin if you're not already doing so?

Why Babysitting Is an Ideal Job for Teenage Twins

- When they first start babysitting and may feel insecure about their abilities, they can babysit together to keep each other company and not feel as if they're tackling this huge responsibility all alone. Parents will be happy to get a "two-for-one" babysitting deal, and the twins can split up when they're older and feel more confident in their abilities.

- They give parents in need of a sitter more options. If one twin is unavailable, the other may be free. Or, if one twin accepts a job and another commitment comes up, his twin may be able to assume the babysitting job.

- Twins can recommend each other for other jobs. If Mrs. Smith is having one twin babysit on a particular night and her friend Mrs. Jones also needs a sitter for the same party, the sitter can recommend her twin!

- Twin babysitters are a bonus for large families or groups of children from multiple families because they can babysit together and better meet the needs of a large group of children. This also holds true if they're babysitting for children who may have difficult temperaments. It's easier to have patience with such a child when there are two caretakers.

- They have a shared occupation that they can talk to each other about and, especially, swap tips and concerns. If Susie had a particularly tough time getting her charge to take his nap, her sister Sarah may have come across the same problem with one of her jobs and can pass along what worked for her to Susie.

- Twins sometimes grow up interacting with fewer children because they always have each other as playmates, so a job working with children gives them the opportunity to experience what it's like to be around others.

Intriguing Twins
DEBRA AND LISA GANZ

Identical twins Debbie and Lisa Ganz have become media darlings with their "multiple" enterprises! With actor Tom Berenger (not a twin), they opened the first ever Twins Restaurant in New York City. It was staffed entirely by identical twins who worked the same shifts. Every night the restaurant was visited by a seemingly endless stream of twin customers. If one twin waitperson was ill and unable to come to work, his or her twin was also told to stay at home. Unfortunately, if one twin got fired, the other got the same treatment! Customers who were multiples got to sign the twin guest book, had their pictures taken for the wall, and received two-for-one drinks. (And, yes, triplets got three-for-one and quadruplets got four-for-one!) The restaurant sported lots of things in pairs, including double door knobs, double light fixtures, and double bar stools.

Debbie and Lisa are also the founders of Twins Talent, a referral service and talent agency that deals exclusively with multiples. They cast twins for movies, commercials, television shows, and special events. The Ganz girls themselves have appeared in more than six hundred television programs, radio shows, commercials, and other productions. Debbie and Lisa have also published a gift book called *The Book of Twins: A Celebration in Words and Pictures,* which includes pictures and essays about twins, and even a twins calendar. The Ganz girls are a living testament that twins are "in"!

When Twin Teens Mature Physically at Different Rates

Teens are naturally insecure about their changing bodies, but this physical transformation can be especially acute if they are early or late bloomers. Kids who develop early may feel embarrassed by their large breasts or deep voice when the other kids in the class still look and sound like children. Conversely, teens who develop late may feel inferior if they're much smaller than their classmates or haven't gotten their "curves" yet. This problem can be especially acute when twins mature at different rates. Of course, this is more common for fraternal twins, but it's not unheard of for identical twins to experience it, too, for various reasons. One twin being seen as more socially acceptable can drive a wedge between the two. The less developed twin may resent her twin's maturity, while the more developed twin may feel she is in an awkward position between defending her twin from critics and earning acceptance from her peers. Same-sex twins often have the most difficulty with differing maturational rates, as they're more likely to be compared.

If your twins are physically maturing at different rates, you can help out by stressing each child's individual strengths. For example, if Jason is maturing more slowly than his twin Aaron, you might want to give Jason some extra encouragement and praise for his skill in playing soccer. Teach your twins that many other qualities are worthy of praise besides physical traits. Most of all, encourage your twins to be understanding of each other's differences. Don't be alarmed if they grow apart a little during this time of change. This is natural and no cause for concern, unless they develop a true dislike for each other or show signs of serious emotional problems. In time, their physical development will "catch up" and they'll find common ground again.

Points to Ponder

Have your twins started going through puberty yet? What signs have you seen, both emotional and physical?

Are your twins maturing at the same or different rates? In what ways are they different?

What unique strengths and talents do each of your twins have that you can emphasize to help them feel good about themselves?

Marriage Survival 101

Raising adolescents can be a strain on any marriage, but when you have two teens in the house, the challenges may be magnified. When your multiples become teenagers—and begin *acting* like teenagers—this can frequently cause stress and strain on your marriage. This may be a time when differences in parenting styles really come to a head. If you were a shy teenager and regret many of the opportunities you missed because of it, you may strongly encourage your twins to be as social as possible. Your spouse, on the other hand, may feel that your adolescents need more structure during this time. He may not be ready for the twins to be out on their own, and so he reins them in. When your twins realize these differences of opinion, they may start playing you against each other. They'll complain to you if their father wants them to stay in for the evening, and you'll be placed in the uncomfortable situation of overruling your husband if you don't agree with him or making your children angry at you if you do agree. It's a no-win situation. The household may be filled with more tension as arguments ensue. Sometimes the household may be split in half as one teen identifies more with her father while the other sides with her mother.

It sounds cliché, but communication is extremely important during this time. First, you and your spouse need to sit down together and iron out the ground rules. It's important to listen to each other's viewpoints and reasons for decisions. Learning about each other's upbringing and experiences will help you understand your partner's parenting style. See if you can compromise on certain issues. For instance, perhaps you can agree that your children may go out one night a week, but it must be with someone you know and approve of, and they must be home by 11:00 P.M. Once you and your spouse have ironed out your differences, have a family meeting. (Don't call it a "family meeting," though, or the kids will groan and tune you out!) Let your teens know the new rules and that you, as the parents, are in agreement in enforcing them. If a situation arises that has not been discussed, tell your twins that you will discuss it with your spouse and return to them later with an answer.

Also, don't forget that you are more than parents; you are a couple, too! Don't sacrifice all of your time by catering to the children and running them around. Make it a tradition that a certain night of the week is for the two of you to go to dinner alone. Take a long weekend away together while the twins stay with friends or relatives. And don't be afraid to let your twins see you being affectionate with each other. They may roll their eyes and groan when they see you kiss, but you're ultimately setting a great example for them of what a marriage should be like. Don't neglect your marital relationship because you're too busy with your children's concerns. A healthy relationship for you means, ultimately, a healthier family for all. Teens are extraordinarily adept at sensing problems in their parents' marriage, no matter how much you try to hide them. And, when there's tension between the two of you, it's bound to affect your children as well. If you find you're not enjoying family life anymore, seek professional help, not only for the sake of your marriage, but also for the well-being of your children.

Points to Ponder

Do you and your spouse differ in your parenting styles? In what ways? Is one of you more a "softie" while the other's more of a disciplinarian?

How do you settle differences in opinion with your partner when it comes to discipline issues? Have you been able to work out compromises on those issues on which you disagree?

How have child-rearing issues affected your marriage now that your twins are teenagers? Do you think you need to spend more time focused on improving your marriage? How would you like to do this?

Is It Too Late to Join a Multiples Group?

Although it's true that parents of multiples are more likely to join support groups when their children are young, don't feel that you won't fit in just because your twins are now teens. First of all, think about what a great mentor you could be to the parents of young twins. You've gone through many experiences with your multiples already, so your wisdom could be invaluable to other parents! Or, have you thought about forming a group of your own for parents of older multiples? There are plenty of parents just like you who are dealing with the pressures of parenting teens times two. Advertise for members in the paper and pass the word at your children's school and religious organization. An informal meeting of five or six parents would be perfect. Finally, if you don't have the time or inclination to meet, look for online chat rooms. For example, www.about.com has a forum for the parents of teenage multiples. Be persistent. You should be able to find or create the support group you need.

Points to Ponder

....

Do you ever wish you had another parent who is raising teenage twins to talk to?

Do you feel that raising teenage twins is different from raising teenage singletons?

Do you belong to a multiples group? If not, why not? Have you thought about joining one or creating your own?

Birthday Parties for Adolescent Twins

Not all adolescents want the attention that comes with a birthday party, so be sure to check with your twins before making plans. Allow them to celebrate their birthdays in their own way. If one wants a party and the other doesn't, respect their wishes. Perhaps the "non-party" kid would prefer just to have a friend spend the night or to go to the movies. Also, make sure to take precautions to keep birthday parties under control, such as limiting the number of kids invited, making sure all invitees are well known to the family, having lots of adult supervision, locking away any alcohol, and limiting the party to one area of the house. Following are some fun suggestions for teen and tween parties.

Twins Tips
GREAT PARTY IDEAS FOR TEENS

Music Party: Rent or buy a karaoke machine and video games that incorporate dancing, like "Dance Dance Revolution." Play music videos on TV and plaster the walls with posters of popular groups and singers. Hold a talent show and award winners with CDs, gift cards for music downloads, and posters.

Jewelry Party: Girls especially love this idea. Buy lots of beads and materials to make necklaces, earrings, and bracelets. Be sure to pick up plenty of wire cutters, scissors, string, etc. Have jewelry patterns available or hire someone to give a lesson!

Sports Party: This can be done in many ways. Arrange for a party at a rock climbing facility or a skate park. Rent some court space at a sports arena, park, or YMCA. Or set up sporting activities in your yard: a volleyball court, swimming, croquet, a baseball game. You could even take the kids to a sporting event, like a baseball or basketball game.

Movie Party: Have lots of teen-favorite movies on hand. And encourage the kids to create movies amongst themselves with video cameras and show them at the end of the party. Let your twins give "Twins Choice" awards for the best movies. Decorate the party space with movie posters, and serve popcorn, candy, and nachos.

Luau Party: Decorate your house in a tropical theme. Lead a limbo game and hire an instructor to teach guests the hula! Make smoothies to drink and serve pineapple pizza. Encourage guests to dress in grass skirts and flowered shirts, and hand out leis as party favors.

Pizza Party: What kid doesn't like pizza? Pass out pre-made mini crusts and let each guest make his or her own pizza. Provide lots of choices for toppings. Yum, yum! Or head on down to the pizza parlor for dinner and video games.

Video Game Party: Rent or borrow various video game systems (PlayStation, Nintendo, GameCube, etc.) and set up gaming stations throughout the house. Make sure you have plenty of popular games available. Award prizes to the winners!

Costume Party: Pick a theme and request that guests come in costume. A renaissance theme is always fun! If it's a co-ed party, have guests dress as the opposite sex. Ask guests to dress as their favorite celebrity, cartoon character, monster, or rock star. Pick a decade with fun clothing styles, such as the 1950s or 1970s. Give prizes for the most creative costumes.

Bowling Party: Many bowling alleys have evenings tailored especially for teens, complete with laser lights, disco balls, and popular music. Check with your local bowling alleys to see if they have a party package or a teen night!

Beauty Party: Girls may enjoy a night of beauty! Arrange for someone to come to the house to give manicures and pedicures. Load up on the makeup and hairstyling supplies and let the girls work on each other's faces and hair. Tell the girls to bring their favorite outfits and have a fashion show!

Points to Ponder

How do your twins feel about having birthday parties now that they're teens? Do they agree or disagree on party plans?

What ideas do you have for great teen parties?

If one or both twins prefer not to have a birthday party, how will they cele-brate instead?

Heading Off to College: Together or Apart?

In most cases, twins attend the same high school (even if they're not always in the same classes), so the decision as to whether to attend the same university or not is a major one. This could be the first time that your multiples have been separated for a substantial period of time! Some twins can't imagine being apart and don't even consider applying to separate schools. Other twins realize that they'll eventually have to take different paths in life and consider this the perfect opportunity to begin that process. After being "roommates" all of their lives, they may feel strongly that they are ready for a break from each other and want to live as singletons. Of course, if they have chosen different career paths, they may be forced to attend different schools if they can't find one that offers both programs.

Some parents may pressure their twins to go in one direction or another. For instance, they may encourage their twins to attend the same college so that they can be roommates and not need to worry about rooming with a stranger who might not be compatible. There's security in going away to college with someone by your side. And if twins have the same classes, they may be able to cut down on costs by sharing the same books and supplies! Other parents may feel that their twins have always been a little too close and now want to encourage them to separate. And twins might find it a refreshing change not always being known as one of "the twins." Often, if they go to separate schools, they may not even let many people know that they have a twin! This is natural.

Going to college is a huge commitment for your twins, so it's generally important to let them make the decision for themselves as to whether to be together or apart. If you insist that they separate against their wishes, they could end up dropping out of college because they're miserable apart. Conversely, if you insist they stay together, they may resent you for the decision and miss out on a great opportunity to really discover themselves as individuals.

Of course, sometimes we make plans—and life has other things in store. For instance, both twins may apply to the same school, but only one gets accepted. This can obviously cause pain and jealousy between them. In the long run, though, a situation like this may turn out for the best. Your twins may both be upset about this at first, but then find out later that it works out fine as they adapt to their new schools and realize that each one is a perfect fit for their particular personalities. They may also find that they enjoy being away from the competitiveness that they engaged in at high school.

Financially, though, attending the same college may be beneficial. Some colleges offer discounts when two family members attend at the same time. And certain schools even offer scholarships for twins. Search the internet or contact your local Parents of Multiples group for information about scholarships for college-bound multiples.

Heading off to college is always a big step for teens and their parents, whether they're singletons or multiples. So, parents of twins must be doubly sensitive to their children's separation anxiety, not only due to being apart from their parents, but also from the possibility of leaving their twin. This can also be an incredibly rewarding time for you as you see your twins blossom on their own and further develop into the individuals they were created to be.

Points to Ponder

Do you think your twins should attend the same college or different colleges? Why?

Do your twins want to go to college together or attend different colleges? Why?

If your twins attend different colleges, how do you think they will handle the adjustment? How will you handle it as their parent?

Intriguing Twins
MARGUERITE AND MARJORIE MAITLAND

When identical twins Marguerite and Marjorie were seventy-five years old, they saw a TV program that featured a wealthy man who used his money to establish a foundation for students at the high school he once attended. For any student who stayed away from drinking, drugs, and smoking, he paid their tuition for college or vocational school. Marguerite and Marjorie were retired and had limited resources, but they were determined to come up with a similar plan. After some brainstorming, they created a program called Project 2001 Plus to encourage students to be drug free in their small Illinois town. Soon, support was gathered from several area churches and members were recruited to run the program. Kids were introduced to the program's benefits in the third grade. They were told that if they stayed away from harmful substances throughout their school years, they would be given $2,000 toward college expenses. The twins held all kinds of fundraisers, such as bake sales, and solicited grants and donations. They also made a special effort to get to know the kids they were encouraging by arranging picnics and play dates with them. Parents were also educated about how to help their kids stay away from drugs and alcohol. On May 20, 2001, the first graduating class was scheduled to receive their scholarships. Unfortunately, fundraising efforts had come up short and only $1,000 was raised for each graduate. Marguerite and Marjorie felt bad that they hadn't kept their promise, but the kids didn't seem to mind; they were still thrilled to get half the money. Amazingly, a short time later, a former student from the same high school died and left $119,000 to the program. The twins were able to give the additional $1,000 to each graduate, plus begin saving for the next class! The sisters continue to run the program even though they're nearly ninety years old. Provisions have been made for the program to go on after their deaths. What an amazing legacy!

Precious Memories

Remember when your twins . . .

- actually thought it was cute to dress alike?
- gave double hugs and kisses at the drop of a hat?
- were "riding in style" in their double stroller?
- smiled at you in the rearview mirror from their car seats in the back of the car?
- wanted matching bikes for Christmas? (Now it's matching cars!)
- played music that didn't hurt your ears?
- liked you to read bedtime stories to them?
- weren't embarrassed to bathe or sleep at the same time?
- actually liked sharing a room?
- could both fit into your arms together?
- would let you pick out their clothes and hairstyles?
- loved to help around the house?
- could scale a baby gate in two seconds flat?
- got excited when you came to their school?
- held hands with each other?
- were happy with gifts as long as they were Barbies or Power Rangers?
- got all kinds of attention for being twins?
- were born? (The best day of your life!)

Don't you miss the old days?

They *Do* Grow Up!

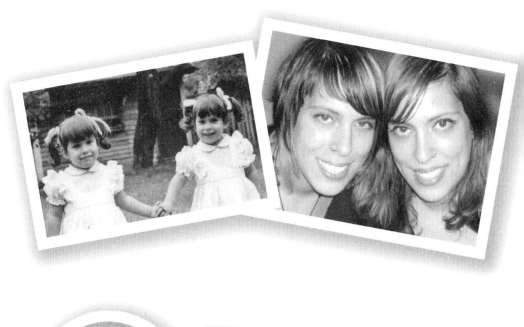

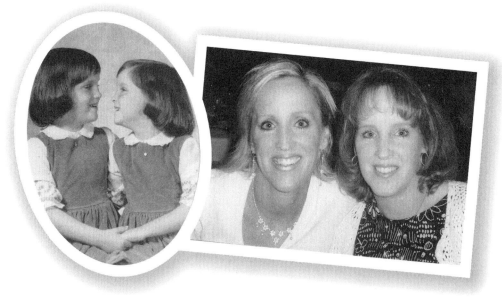

A Final Word from the Author

Dear Parents,

I hope by now you've gotten the message that our families are very special! You and I have been chosen for the privileged role of being the parent of multiples. Sure, we have double (or triple) the challenges of most families, but we also have even more joy, fun, and excitement in our lives than singleton parents. Honestly, doesn't the thought of life without multiples now just seem so dull?

My hope is that this book not only provided some guidance and support for you as you raise your twins (or triplets or more), but also put a smile on your face, a chuckle in your heart, and a belly laugh in, well, your belly! It was my intention to make *It's Twins!* not only helpful, but entertaining as well.

Parents of multiples always seem to be a friendly bunch, willing to share the wisdom they've gained over their many years of double trouble and double blessings. If reading this book prompted you to think of some great stories of your own, or some useful advice or tips for other parents of multiples, I'd love to hear from you. Please visit my Web site at www.susanheim.com and drop me a line. It's possible you could be featured in my next book!

And be sure to send copies of this book to the other parents of multiples in your life. As you know, they can never get enough help!

In conclusion, I'd like to present one more collection of advice written by mother of triplets, Nancy Johnson. She did a great job of summing up the most important lessons that every parent of multiples should learn. Enjoy!

Many blessings,
Susan M. Heim

Twins Tale

THINGS I'VE LEARNED AS A MOM OF MULTIPLES
Nancy Johnson

1. Making them wait teaches them patience.
2. It's okay if they share the same spoon or drink from the same bottle.
3. It *is* possible to breastfeed triplets!
4. Learning how to take turns teaches them a valuable life skill.
5. A mom of multiples *does* have enough love to go around.
6. They can all bathe in the same bath water.
7. Thrift shops are a good thing.
8. Let your kids teach *you* some things.
9. When one gets sick, you can almost bet the other(s) will, too (see #2).
10. You will *always* have concern for their well-being.
11. Birthdays are real causes for celebration.
12. Dads will surprise you—just when you think they don't have a clue.
13. Dads really *can't* read your mind, so tell them when you need their help.
14. Just when you've figured out your multiples' schedule, it changes!
15. It's okay to feel sorry for people who aren't parents of multiples.
16. It's okay to feel sorry for *yourself* because you are a parent of multiples.

17. Multiples learn how to count and measure sooner than their singleton peers. ("She has more juice than I have!" "His cookie is bigger than mine!")

18. Sometimes, if you can't laugh, it's okay to cry!

19. You will wish, more than once, that you could be cloned.

20. It is truly much more important to cuddle and love your babies than it is for you to have a house that is always clean.

21. Miraculously, after you have finally accepted the fact that you will never be able to sleep again, your babies *will* sleep through the night (although you may not believe it when it actually happens).

22. It is okay to switch pediatricians if you decide that yours just doesn't understand multiples.

23. A mother's instinct is usually right.

24. It's okay if, when you finally go out *alone* with your spouse, you do nothing but talk about the kids.

25. Your life will be forever changed when you become the parent of multiples, but that is a *good* thing.

26. Teach your children early what a "scholarship" is—they are going to need it!

27. You will invariably have at least one picky eater.

28. Schedules are good, but so is flexibility.

29. Teach your children how to spend, save, and donate.

30. Keep a journal and make daily notes about how you felt and what you and your babies did. Your children will find this very entertaining when they are older.

31. Don't ever forget how special your family really is.

32. You aren't superhuman. Accept help when it is offered.

33. Learn to be as independent as possible so that when there is no help, you can handle it.

34. Super-center stores are great. They often have multi-kid shopping carts, you can run several errands in one stop, and there is plenty of stimulation for your kids. (You may also find other grownups to talk to!)

35. Competition can be a useful thing. Think potty training, getting good grades, etc.

36. Always be prepared with more diapers, toys, snacks, drinks, clothes, etc., than you think you will need.

37. Parents of multiples are often more creative than parents of singletons.

38. Introduce your children to vegetables from an early age.

39. Cook with your children. Once you get past the stress and mess, you will reap the rewards.

40. Your kids will eventually learn about McDonald's. You can't fight it.

41. Good parents do make mistakes.

42. It's okay if your little boy is proud of the fact that he can "walk real good" in your high-heeled shoes.

43. Band-Aids, icepacks, and kisses fix a lot of things.

44. Sing and dance with your kids, even if you can't carry a tune in a bucket and have two left feet.

45. You will never find the perfect time to discuss "the birds and the bees"; it finds *you*.

46. If you think you've done a great job childproofing your home, think again!

47. One of your multiples will eventually dial 911 and hang up.

48. Eventually, you will be able to make it through a meal without someone having to go to the bathroom as soon as hot food is served.

49. Pretend you don't hear them when people ask if you are going to have more children.

50. Choose your battles—there will be lots of them!

51. When your multiples are at each other's throats, remember those times when they held hands, tied each other's shoes, and played nicely together.

52. Teach your children early the value of family.

Meet the Parents

I'd like to extend a huge "thank you" to all of the parents of multiples who so generously shared their stories and advice for this book. This section will let you read a little more about them, and if they've included their e-mail address, feel free to contact them and let them know how their material helped you. I could never have written this book without their extensive feedback and contributions. Applause, applause!

Rebecca Adamitis is an aspiring writer. She holds a bachelor's degree in theater arts and has established a career in the graphic arts and printing industry. Rebecca is married and lives in a suburb of Chicago, Illinois, with her preschool-aged son and boy/girl toddler twins. She can be contacted via e-mail at roocrewma@yahoo.com regarding her experiences with pregnancy complications, prematurity, and NICU stays, as well as the parenting of multiples and Sensory Integration Syndrome.

Bette Ade and her husband Carl have been married for forty-nine years. They have three daughters, three sons-in-law, and eight "grands" (four girls and four boys, ranging in age from seven to twenty-five). Bette is a former airline hostess and her husband is a retired airline captain. She has owned her own business, *Creations from Bette's Belfrey*, for more than twenty-five years, designing and making baby and gift accessories. She sells to specialty shops all over the U.S. Bette is the founder and past president of Texas Mothers of Multiples, as well as a past president of Dallas Mothers of Twins and Triplets Club, both support groups for parents of multiple birth children.

Mary Brauer has written numerous twin-related articles that have appeared in local newspapers and *TWINS* magazine. She lives in Massachusetts with her husband and fraternal twin sons. Mary can be reached at brauer_mary@yahoo.com.

Sage de Beixedon Breslin, PhD, is a licensed psychologist who specializes in personal transformation. She is also senior editor for Zur Institute, an online CEU provider. Sage has authored chapters and articles on a wide variety of topics and has a book on the market. *Lovers & Survivors: Living with and Loving a Sexual Abuse Survivor* is available for purchase through RDR Publishers or through Dr. Breslin at Sage@HealingHeartCenter.org or www.healingheartcenter.org.

Michelle Brouillette is a full-time wife, mother, and college student majoring in early childhood education. She has been married to her husband Kerry for sixteen years and they have three children. Sean is eight years old and is the older brother of twin sisters, Abigail and Hanna, who are five years old.

Cheryl Oberbeck Burns is a writer and poet. She lives in Palo Alto, California, with her husband and twin boys, Jack and Chase.

Holly Caldwell, a stay-at-home mother of six-year-old twins and a three-year-old, promotes reading to children as an independent Usborne book consultant. Before being put on bed rest at twenty weeks with her twin pregnancy, Holly created employee publications for a religious publisher. Holly's wonderful husband, Jay, is an excellent example of how hands-on a twin dad should be.

Lorelei Capuzzi and her husband Peter, a United States Marine, are currently stationed in Hawaii, where they live with their eighteen-month-old twin boys, Rocco and Peter. They are expecting their third child in early 2007.

Lainie Ceasar was a fourth grade teacher for eight years before she and her husband were blessed with twin boys. She has temporarily left her profession to stay home with her year-and-a-half-old boys, Max and Zack. She and her family reside in Rockland County, New York. Lainie can be reached at lceasar@optonline.net.

Michele Christian resides in Abington, Massachusetts, and is a mother of three children: one boy and twin girls.

Tara Coleran has been married to Ted for four years. They are best friends and work well as a team to raise three small children. Their lives changed forever when they found out at seven weeks of pregnancy that they would be having twins. Their oldest child, Brett, was only fifteen months old at the time! Tara is a survivor of HELLP Syndrome, which caused her twins to be six weeks premature but with no complications.

Lisa Crystal is a northern California writer who chronicles the joys and challenges of raising children who arrive singly and in pairs. She draws infinite inspiration from her identical twin sons, whom she home-schools, and her teenage daughter. Lisa's book, *Mother's Little Helper: First-Year Sanity Savers the "Experts" Won't Tell You*, is due out in 2007. She welcomes reader comments at www.lisacrystal.blogspot.com.

Holly Engel-Smothers lives in Buckner, Maryland. She has had several books and articles published. Holly has been an educator since 1990, specializing in reading. Holly and her husband Dan enjoy the love, activity, and surprises that come with raising their identical twin girls, age seven, and singleton daughter, age four.

Pat Enriquez has been a travel agent for more than thirty years and works at South Mountain Travel in West Orange, New Jersey. She moved to Mexico City with a girlfriend when she was twenty-three years old and met her husband Mannie. They have been happily married ever since! Their identical twin daughters, Nicole and Janine, were born in 1979. In 1987, her husband's job transferred them to Germany, where they all lived for almost two years. Since they had their children two at a time, Pat and her husband decided not to have any more, but they did adopt twin cats named Misty and Ebony (which, thankfully, they didn't have to send to college!).

Joanne Higgins Ensign is the daughter of a fraternal twin. She is a seasoned first-grade teacher and a budding writer. Joanne has also contributed to a *TWINS* magazine project. She lives in beautiful San Diego County, California, with her husband, and is the proud mother of three children: fraternal twin daughters and a son. She can be reached at joannehensign@yahoo.com.

Marla Feldman lives in a quiet neighborhood with her husband of nineteen years and their three children. An elementary school teacher for twelve years, Marla can now be found working part-time in both her synagogue's religious school and preschool. She enjoys being home with her family.

Cindy Ferraino and her husband Jeff live in New Jersey with their three children: identical twin daughters and a son.

Adarezza Ferrer graduated as a physician and surgeon from the University of San Carlos de Guatemala. Mother of a five-year-old girl and fourteen-month-old twin girls, Adarezza lives with her husband and daughters in Pleasant Hill, California.

Kristy Fitzgerald, a former special education teacher, is now happy to be at home with her children. She is a part-time nursing student and hopes to become an NICU nurse. Kristy lives in Lompoc, California, with her husband Scott, daughter Sydney (four years old), and twin sons Anthony and Alex (two-and-a-half years old).

John C. Flewellen is an aspiring poet. John has written numerous poems about his family and poems for his friends. He has been married for twenty-eight years and has five children. His twelve-year-old identical twin sons both have Crohn's/colitis and have inspired many of his poems. His e-mail address is fotplus3@aol.com.

Nicole M. Gates-Hulbert is a Joliet, Illinois, native. She currently resides in Memphis, Tennessee. She is married to Darrick Hulbert and is the proud mother of four daughters: Yolanda (sixteen), Savanna (six), and twins Brooklyn and Bheanna (one). Nicole is a recent member of the Chicago Jaycees, Will Mother of Twins Club, Chicago Festival Association, Will County Reading Association, International Reading Association, Character Counts Coalition, and Parents as Teachers. She is a current member of Memphis Mothers of Multiples and Memphis Mocha Moms. Nicole serves as cofounder of W.O.M.A.N./S.I.S.T.A.S., Joliet/Memphis Heartwarmers, and Seeds of Success. She is owner of More than a Memory Event Planners and Delicious Wishes Confectionary. Nicole's motto: "Reach for the Moon and You'll Land among the Stars"!

Lisa Henshaw is the mother of boy/girl toddler twins. She is married and lives in Tampa, Florida. She can be reached at lhenshaw@tampabay.rr.com.

Lori Iventosch-James and her husband, Fred James, live in Los Gatos, California, with their fraternal twin boys, Gabriel and Daniel James. Life with the boys is never boring!

Anne K. Jacobs, PhD, is a clinical child psychologist currently working as a researcher with the Terrorism and Disaster Center of the National Child Traumatic Stress Network. Her professional publications focus on psychological first aid and evaluating treatments for children with serious emotional disturbances, developmental psychopathology, research methods, and bullying. Anne lives with her husband, Noel (also a clinical child psychologist), and twin daughters, Sarah and Keegan. You can contact her at azerg@sbcglobal.net.

Denice Aldrich Jobe has written essays and features that have appeared in *The Washington Post, AAUW Outlook, Brevity,* and *Preemie.* She also writes fiction and is currently at work on a novel. In June 2003, she gave birth to twin boys after spending eleven weeks in the hospital on bed rest.

Nancy Johnson is originally from Goshen, New York, but has lived in central Florida since 1984. Nancy has her BS in Business Economics and works for a pharmaceutical company. She is also a licensed realtor. Nancy is married and the mother of triplets.

Leslie Kelley-Genson graduated from Virginia's Radford University before getting her Master of Social Work degree from Virginia Commonwealth University. She lives with her husband, identical four-year-old twin sons Seth and Ben, and new daughter Emma outside Charlottesville, Virginia, where she works as a marketing specialist for the city's Parks and Recreation Department. She can be reached at lesliekelley@earthlink.net.

Cheryl Maguire received her bachelor's and master's degrees in counseling psychology from Boston College. She has worked in many different settings as a counselor for children and their families. Cheryl is married and lives in East Bridgewater, Massachusetts, with her boy/girl toddler twins. She enjoys being a stay-at-home mom.

Terri Mobbs is a wife and stay-at-home mom to a daughter and twin boys, one of whom has delays due to Twin to Twin Transfusion Syndrome. She is an active volunteer at her church and local twins club. She currently resides in LaVergne, Tennessee.

Nancy Molter is a proud mother of three preschoolers. She and her husband have five-and-a-half-year-old twin daughters adopted from Stavropol, Russia. They also have a son who is four. The children fill their days with laughter and laundry! They reside in Cincinnati, Ohio. For any questions about international adoption or advice on keeping your sanity with three babies in diapers, feel free to contact Nancy at nancymolter3@aol.com.

Pam Pace is a cofounder of Keeping Pace with Multiple Miracles, a nonprofit support organization for families who have or who are expecting twins, triplets, or quadruplets in Massachusetts. Pam is the mother of five beautiful children: triplets Brittany, Brandi, Stephen (twelve), Bailey (eleven), and Benjamin (ten). Pam has been supporting and facilitating support group meetings for multiples for the past eleven years. Pam also breastfed all of her children, including the triplets. She is a La Leche League leader and is passionate about supporting and helping other mothers of multiples have positive breastfeeding experiences. Pam was put on bed rest during her high-risk pregnancy and delivered her multiples at only twenty-nine weeks. She speaks at conferences and is sought after for her multiple birth experience. Pam has written for various parenting publications, including *TWINS* magazine. As an advocate for multiple birth families, Pam has met with several agencies, such as the DPH, March of Dimes, Early Intervention, MSPCC, CTF, and the United Way to determine how multiples in Massachusetts can be better supported. Pam is a member of MOST, The Triplet Connection, and the National Organization of Mothers of Twins Club. Pam has been married to her husband, Stephen, for seventeen years and resides in Bridgewater. She can be reached at keepingpace.multiplemiracles@verizon.net and www.keepingpace.org.

Lisa Clifton Philbrook is a navy wife and a stay-at-home mom. Lisa lives in Pensacola, Florida, with her family: a teenage daughter, a ten-year-old son, and identical toddler twins.

Sherri R. Polhemus is a mother of fraternal twin girls who lives with her husband and children in Las Vegas, Nevada. She is a student, volunteer, scrapbooker, and homemaker who enjoys writing in her spare time. She can be contacted at sherrirp@earthlink.net.

Laurel Hemmig Porterfield, a writer and mother of three, tries to maintain an attitude of gratitude every day.

Roxy Ranelli was born near Pittsburgh, Pennsylvania, twenty-eight years ago. She has since completed a BS in Special Education from Slippery Rock University and an MS in Humanities and Organizational Management. A former manager, she is currently "managing" three beautiful babies!

Mary Reeves is first and foremost a wife of eleven years and a mother of identical twin girls born in November 1998. The family lives in Aurora, Colorado. In the "outside" world, Mary has the job title of Program Manager at the Association of periOperative Registered Nurses (AORN), which she enjoys very much. Mary is also active in the Parent Teacher Community Organization (PTCO) at her girls' elementary school. She is the secretary of the Executive Board and is enjoying learning the ropes of the PTCO.

Kim M. Rich is the author of the memoir *Johnny's Girl* (Alaska Northwest Books, 1999), which chronicles her growing up in Alaska's underworld with her father, a professional gambler who was murdered when Kim was fifteen. In 1995, Hallmark Entertainment adapted the story into a movie starring Treat Williams. Kim also contributed an essay for the anthology, *Our Alaska,* edited by Mike Doogan (Epicenter Press, 2001) and *The Day My Father Died*, edited by Diana Ajjan (Running Press, 1994). Kim's short story, "Terminal," appeared in *The Mysterious North,* edited by Dana Stabenow (Penguin, 2003). Kim began her career with the *Anchorage Daily News*. She has an MFA in Creative Writing from Columbia University. In 1997, Perseverance Theater in Juneau was awarded a National Endowment for the Arts grant for the stage adaptation of *Johnny's Girl*. Kim wrote the adaptation, and the play had its world premiere that year. Kim currently works as a screenwriter and novelist, and is a writer in residence at Alaska Pacific University, where she also teaches writing.

Christine Scheeler, married for sixteen years to her wonderful husband Mike, is now a proud stay-at-home mother to her boy/girl twins born in October 2005. Prior to becoming a full-time, hands-on mom, Christine was a technical trainer. Currently, her spare time is focused on operating her successful PhotographyMom.com portrait studio.

Lynne Sella's career as an author was launched when she began making up stories for the sole purpose of entertaining her twin daughters. Hooked by the joy of writing, she has written children's stories, humorous anecdotes about living with twins, a romance set in Mendocino, and a series of stories about the misadventures of a female deputy sheriff. She lives with her family in Susanville, California, and dreams of the day when she can make writing her full-time career.

Sherry St. James is a public speaker and freelance writer who specializes in personal essays and customized children's stories for kids with special circumstances. She has three beautiful children of her own, each arriving in an unusual way. Sherry lives in Lawrence, Kansas, and can be reached at sherry123e@aol.com.

Donna Sullivan is a graduate of the University of Alabama. Her short story, "My Mother the Fortune Teller," has been included in the book *Twice the Love: Stories of Inspiration for Families . . . with Twins, Multiples, and Singletons* (available through *TWINS* magazine). She is married and has preschool-age identical twin girls and a toddler son. She lives in Springfield, Virginia.

Erika Tremper is a happily married, proud mother of six-year-old twin girls. She works as a business systems analyst and lives in Hillsborough, New Jersey, where she finds time to read a lot and to write a little. You can contact her at etremper@patmedia.net.

Jason Westcott is a power tool salesman. He is married and lives in Plainfield, Illinois, with his twin boys.

Deanne Whiteley, a former Human Resources Generalist, is now a stay-at-home mum, job search instructor, and newsletter feature writer. An active volunteer, she works as a pregnancy/newborn hotline advisor and area representative for the WSCMMOTA twins club. Deanne is also a mentor for the Parent Connection at Beth Israel Deaconess Medical Center, where she provides support and advice for first-time families with multiples or singleton newborns. She is an avid traveler and has lived in Australia, Japan, England, France, and America, although she calls Australia home. Deanne now lives in Boston, Massachusetts, with her cheeky twin toddlers, wonderful husband Chris, and American Eskimo Shiraz. Deanne can be contacted at deannewhiteley@yahoo.com.au.

Index

I

J

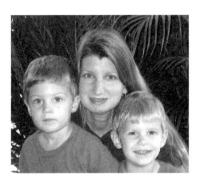

About the Author

Susan M. Heim is a writer and editor who specializes in parenting, multiples, and women's issues. She enjoys developing proposals and manuscripts with many high-profile authors. Before starting her own writing and editing business, Susan was a senior editor for the best-selling *Chicken Soup for the Soul* series. She is the coauthor of *Oh, Baby! 7 Ways a Baby Will Change Your Life the First Year* (Hampton Roads) and the author of *Twice the Love: Stories of Inspiration for Families . . . with Twins, Multiples, and Singletons,* published in conjunction with *TWINS* magazine. Her writing has appeared in many other books and publications.

Susan is a ClubMom parenting expert and writes a multiples column, "Loving and Living with Twins and Multiples," on the Mommies Magazine website. She has a blog, "Susan Heim on Parenting," at www.susanheim.blogspot.com. She is a member of the National Association of Women Writers and the Southeastern Writers Association and holds a degree in business administration from Michigan State University. Susan lives in Florida with her husband Mike and their four sons: Dylan, Taylor, and twins Austen and Caleb. She welcomes all correspondence through her Web site at www.susanheim.com.

Hampton Roads Publishing Company

... for the evolving human spirit

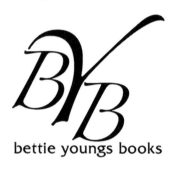

bettie youngs books

Inspiring each other with hope, possibility, and courage.

HAMPTON ROADS PUBLISHING COMPANY
publishes books on a variety of subjects,
including metaphysics, spirituality,
health, visionary fiction, and other related topics.

For a copy of our latest trade catalog,
call toll-free, 800-766-8009,
or send your name and address to:

HAMPTON ROADS PUBLISHING COMPANY, INC.
1125 STONEY RIDGE ROAD • CHARLOTTESVILLE, VA 22902
E-mail: hrpc@hrpub.com • Internet: www.hrpub.com